HOW

CANCER

Fighting Back With Alternative Methods

By
CHESTER F. GAINES

C & B Publishing
Copyright © 2015 Chester Gaines
All rights reserved.
Email: chestergaines@aol.com

How I Beat Cancer: Fighting Back With Alternative Methods

Written	Chester Gaines
Edited & Typography	Trish Geran
Cover Design	Chester Gaines & Trish Geran

This book is intended to be an educational tool to acquaint the reader with alternative methods of preventing and treating cancer. My hope is to improve your well-being and to better understand, evaluate, and choose the appropriate course of treatment. The methods described in this book are for the most part alternative methods, by definition, and many of them have not been investigated and/or approved by any government or regulatory agency. National, state, and local laws vary regarding the use and application of many of the treatments that are discussed. Accordingly, this book should not be substituted for the advice and treatment of a licensed physician or any other health care professional. Pregnant women are urged to consult with their physician before using any of these therapies.

I do not claim to be a doctor and therefore I shall not be liable or responsible for the loss, damage, or injury of any person caused or alleged directly or indirectly by the information I have provided. No representation or warranties of any kind are made with regard to completeness or accuracy of the information. Quotations are used as "fair use" to illustrate various points made. Quoted text may be subject to copyright owned by third parties.

Gaines, Chester F.
Bibliography
1. Gaines, Chester F., 1934 -
2. Alternative treatments for prostate cancer
3. Healing prostate cancer naturally
3. Prostate cancer symptoms
4. Economic impact & statistics on cancer in the United States

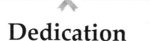

Dedication

This book is dedicated to my family and close friends that I lost to cancer. My aunts Audrey Morrow (breast), Ruby Roach (lung), Bernice Evans (brain), my cousin Bobby Edmunds (prostate), friend Hattie Watts (breast), and many members in my church. Numerous times, I attempted to convince them to try alternative treatments but they were already "sold" on their doctor's advice and rejected my suggestion even after learning that my prostate cancer was in remission. These tender people touched my life in so many ways and to have witnessed them suffer even after receiving chemotherapy, radiation, or surgery, cautioned me even more about the success of traditional medicine and orthodox treatments. It is my desire that the information contained within this book restores the general health of the readers and create confidence to at least try one of these alternative treatments that saved my life and others who are still here to inspire many who continue to suffer.

Acknowledgments

I never would have been able to write and complete this book without the patience of my dear wife Wilma "Bunny." I spent countless hours in my office doing research and writing as she continued to run our business without my assistance.

I would like to thank Dr. Leedell W. Neyland, former professor of History and Dean of College of Arts & Science and interim Vice President at Florida A & M University, for encouraging me to pursue the completion of this project and for introducing me to author/editor, Trish Geran. She was the foundation needed to complete this book and to make sure it was launched in a timely manner.

And mostly, I would like to thank God for restoring my health when cancer came knocking at my door and for giving me the determination to write a story that will hopefully heal others.

Everyone should know that the war on cancer is largely a fraud.

--- Dr. Linus Pauling ---
Chemist, biochemist, peace activist, author, and educator and the recipient of the Nobel Prize in Chemistry and the Nobel Peace Prize.

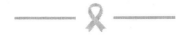

Contents

Notes:
   Bibliographies
   References

Chapter 1

My Reason, My Purpose

In 2000, I was diagnosed with cancer. On February 26th, I had a routine yearly physical which included an EKG, blood tests, and x-rays. I left the doctor's office feeling confident that I would definitely receive my normal "bill of health" stamp. A few days later, his office called and asked if I would come in that following Thursday to go over my tests results. This was an unusual follow up but even so I remained confident things were going to be okay. I was feeling great and I was involved in numerous organizations so I didn't entertain for a second the notion that something was wrong.

At 3:30 p.m., I arrived at the office still feeling overly confident that is until the doctor walked into the room with a grim look on his face. My chest sunk. He said that my PSA (Prostate-Specific Antigen) count was 28 and "when it is that high it is certain you have prostate cancer." I stood stunned from what I had just heard. I didn't know what to say. He then continued, "We just don't know if it is malignant until we get a biopsy." He recommended an appointment with a urologist and asked that I get back with him before making any decisions to the type of treatment suggested.

The biopsy was positive. The Gleason Prostrate Score reported 3.0 with a PSA count of 28. The urologist immediately wanted to schedule me for surgery. He pushed and I pushed back.

I wanted to know about the operation, the possible side effects, and how long it would take to regain my "normal" lifestyle. He said the recovery for an out-patient would be at least six weeks and the worst case scenario was the possibility of incontinence and the inability to have a normal sex life for quite some time. He highly recommended chemotherapy at a later date to make sure the cancer was gone. Suddenly an alarm went off inside my head. I needed to move in another direction and travel down a road I have never been on. I have witnessed too many of my family and church members and close friends and neighbors die from cancer-a devastating disease-after being under the care of their doctor.

In my lifetime, nothing has been more tragic than to watch a healthy person's appearance dwindle down to skin and bones after receiving traditional orthodox medicine (chemotherapy, radiation, surgery). This experience is agonizing and breaks the spirits of families, a crisis I feel is totally unnecessary.

Their deaths were hastened by physicians who practiced the old treatments which do more harm than good. They destroy the immune system more than they heal the body.

My head began to spin from the balancing act I was trying to make sense out of. I began to recall when a cousin was diagnosed with Prostate cancer and decided to have the surgery followed by a series of chemotherapy treatments. The results were devastating. He lost his hair, dropped an enormous amount of weight, and eventually lost his will to live.

Before I was diagnosed, my life would be deemed as "not out of the ordinary" especially for a smoker. Each morning, I would have a cup of coffee and a cigarette, and then pour another cup or sometimes have orange juice instead along with a couple of pieces of bacon. While traveling in my car to work, I would-at times-smoke one or two cigarettes, and when I got to the office, I would pour a third cup of coffee and grab a doughnut which was followed by a cigarette break. For several decades, this was my morning routine.

For lunch, I would order fast food and a soda or maybe even a beer if I was out with a friend and the occasion called for a toast. Afterwards, I would have a smoke before heading back to work.

Three times a week, dinner consisted of a meal that was surrounded around red meat and fried side dishes. For example, the serving of collard greens would be highly seasoned and cooked with animal fat. The flavor was addicting and I enjoyed being the victim.

Later in the evening, I would mix my favorite drink: Canadian whisky with a splash of ginger ale. I would partake in one or two before the eleven o'clock news and afterwards I turned in. On the average, I slept six to seven hours a night. This was my daily routine for several decades.

I was always full of vigor and vitality, a lifestyle I thought was healthy enough to avoid an encounter with what some refer to as the "Big C."

After being diagnosed, I researched medical findings and testimonies on prostate cancer and discovered that certain lifestyle choices heighten the risk. Smoking, a poor diet, and drinking alcohol are known to increase the chances of not only having cancer but possibly a serious chronic condition such as cardiovascular disease, diabetes, or kidney and liver problems. I use to believe that cancer was genetic and that it is a result of "bad luck". I never in a million years thought it would be knocking on my front door awaiting an answer immediately.

However, not all doctors are more interested in making money than bettering the health of their patients. There are good doctors that are dedicated and more interested in your health. I was fortunate; I had a doctor that helped me find an alternative treatment. Most doctors will not tell you about any natural or alternative health therapies and be able to continue practicing medicine. The AMA regulations would advise against such advice.

My doctor was God sent. He introduced me to alternative treatments knowing it was frowned upon in the American Medical Association (AMA) or by colleagues in the medical industry. He could have been labeled a quack or lost his license but instead he gave me my life back and a chance to help others. That was 15 years ago and today I'm here to tell my story.

Chapter 2

Origins of My Alternatives

Cancer is a disease that one dreads to be told they have. After I received my "news", I felt like a judge had sentenced me to death by lethal injection. I recalled how my friends and family members died from this disease within five years from the last day of receiving orthodox treatments, and I remembered reading how 97% of individuals diagnosed with this disease would more than likely die within a year, if not from cancer it would be from chemotherapy, radiation, or surgery, definite destroyers of the immune system. Cancer is the second largest killer in the United States after heart failure and strokes. That's when I realized the odds were not stacked in my favor.

These fears and questions directed me back to my primary care physician who practiced holistic medicine and I was ready to discuss the various alternative methods.

Haelan 951

He recommended Haelan 951, a concentrated soy beverage that was imported from China. A thirty day supply cost $1,200 plus shipping and handling. After drinking eight ounces of Haelan 951 for one month, my PSA count dropped from 28 to 18. The second month it went from 18 to 15. I was somewhat disappointed with this result. I wondered if I was spending too much money for little results, but I was curious what the results would be after taking the treatment for three months. I had a 13 which was only two points lower. I was disappointed. After calculating the costs of taking the Haelan 951 I realized that this alternative method was going to cost me roughly $14,400 a year to get my PSA to normal and that was not guaranteed.

I had spent a total of $3,600 plus shipping with little success. Maybe I was comparing my health with money, but I am not a rich man and an extra $1,200 each month would place a serious dent in my budget. Alternative medicines was not covered under my hospitalization plan and this was going to be a very costly process. If this was the only alternative I had to choose from then I would continue with it. I asked my physician to recommend a treatment that was less costly. He gave me a list of a few and then he suggested I browse the internet and research the various methods.

After I carefully read my findings, the alternative method I was confident would heal my body of cancer was called, HIGH pH THERAPY, using Cesium Chloride. It was proven to kill cancer cells by changing the pH of the body because cancer cannot live in a healthy alkaline body. The cost was approximately $300.00 for a thirty day supply and the results should occur within 30 to 45 days. I decided to give it a try.

High pH Therapy

Eighty-five years ago, a German doctor named Otto Warburg was awarded two Nobel prizes for his theories that stated cancer was caused by a weakened cell respiration due to a lack of oxygen. What this means is that a healthy cell, oxygen, and glucose can move freely across the cell membrane. Oxygen is then used in a healthy cell to burn glucose and create energy. This process is called respiration.

A cancer cell is a normal cell that has mutated and become anaerobic (meaning it can live without oxygen). In order for the cell to survive it has to manipulate the membrane to keep the oxygen out but allow the glucose to enter. In the absence of oxygen the glucose cannot burn and the in order for the cancer cell to survive it must revert back to a more primitive state and generate its energy through a process called fermentation. Since the newly formed (anaerobic) cancer cell cannot be repaired the cell is now out of control and must be destroyed as rapidly as possible. The cancer cell produces lactic acid which causes the cancer to multiply uncontrollably and causes intense pain that is often associated with cancer.

High pH therapy is when the cancer cell readily takes itself to a total of 6 grams of Cesium Chloride (CsCl) daily through its protective outer cell wall. With the absorption of the CsCl there is an uptake of ascorbic and retionic acids, vitamins C and A, zinc and selenium salts which when absorbed on the membrane surface will act as broad and moderately strong electron donors. These compounds help enhance the cancer cell absorb the Cesium ions.

The results are:

- Cancer cells alkaline;
- Intake of glucose is limited into the cell thus starving the cell;
- Lactic acid is neutralized which is what causes the cell to multiply uncontrollably and eventually kills the cell and makes it nontoxic; and
- Fermentation process stops which is a second effect of limiting the glucose which is what creates lactic acid.

Cancer cells are acidic where normal healthy cells are alkaline with a level slightly above 7.4. They become dormant at a pH of 8 to 8.5 and cannot live at this high alkaline level. Eventually they will die.

The pH range is from 0 to 14. Numbers below pH range 7 are considered acid or low range. The range above 7 represents an alkaline or oxygenated condition. In pH Therapy when Cesium is able to enter a cancer cell, it raises the pH or oxygen content of the cell. The cell cannot survive and is absorbed and eliminated by the body.

I discovered that Cesium can raise the pH of cancer cells but in order to get the maximum absorption, Potassium, Vitamin A and C, Salts of Zinc, plus Selenium must be added. Cesium is a naturally occurring mineral with the atomic number 55 on the periodic table of elements. It is nature's most alkaline mineral.

The following are testimonies of people who had successful results using High pH Therapy using Cesium Chloride:

Testimonial 1:

I am a 65 years old and was diagnosed with colon cancer and pancreatic cancer in June of 2012. The doctor gave me no hope because he said pancreatic cancer was a death sentence and there was nothing they could do for me. In August I heard about the high pH therapy for fighting cancer using the Cesium Chloride. I started taking it along with the potassium and other nutrients. In approximately 1 month I passed what I believed to be the colon cancer which looked like a sponge type octopus with legs almost as big as my fist. After 90 days total of being on the Cesium I was examined again and there was no cancer found, pancreatic or otherwise anywhere in my body.

Sharlene J.

Marion, Indiana

Testimonial 2:

My Brother had a large bump on his head and I dragged him against his will to Dr. Thomas who surgically removed it. My brother refused to go back, but the bump started to come back. The lab called it Squamish cell skin cancer but my 60 year old brother refused to believe it. He finally allowed me to order him some Cesium Chloride and potassium and started sipping at the bottles. Yesterday he told me that the bump had just fallen off as he felt it.

Rodney McFarland for James McFarland,

Victorville, California

Testimonial 3:

My daughter had another brain surgery on June 30 at Duke University Hospital in Durham, N.C. It was as successful as we could have hoped for. The pathology report indicated that a major portion of the tumor was already dead. We considered that a miracle! The doctors have recommended further chemotherapy. We have rejected that proposal, and are going with natural healing totally. In that respect, I continue to remember our conversation regarding Cesium solution. I feel that it's been an important part of her therapy.

Many thanks! All the best to you.

Sincerely,

Mildred FrankowskI

Detroit, Michigan

Testimonial 4:

I have had problems with my prostate for years with my PSA numbers registering the following: 4.1 in 1999 2.0 in 2000 11.7 in2001 I started taking the cancer protocol along with the water soluble Cesium and after only 40 days of taking the (minerals) product my PSA count registered.06!! . The product works!

Glenn Schwartz

Pittsburgh, Pennsylvania

Dr. A. Keith Brewer, PhD has proven that Cesium gets into cancer cells when other nutrients cannot. After entering the cell, it makes the cancer cell alkaline which limits the intake of glucose into the cell and eventually starves the cell and neutralizes the lactic acid. The lactic acid is what causes the cell to multiply uncontrollably. Once the lactic acid is neutralized the cell becomes nontoxic which stops the fermentation process.

Cesium Chloride works by making cancer cells highly alkaline, typically 8.0 and above thus killing the cancer cells. Not only does the Cesium kill the cancer cell it immediately stops the metastasis of the cancer and began to shrink any tumor masses within weeks. Without the lactic acid being present there is no pain. Usually, the pain will stop within 12 to 36 hours after starting the Cesium Chloride treatment.

For the sake of my family and friends, I wish I had known about these facts. Although they were under a physician's care they were compromising their immune systems. In other words, their doctors were killing them.

After 30 days on the Cesium Chloride alternative method, the doctor said that the results from my blood test showed a PSA count of less than four. When I heard these miraculous words, I was overwhelmed with joy. I still had more work to do, but at least there was a glimmer of hope in my future.

Side Effects

During my treatment, I experienced minor flu-like symptoms. I had a tingling sensation around my nose and lips which would last about fifteen minutes after ingesting the Cesium Chloride. I was aware that I might experience nausea because it is supposedly a normal reaction of the Cesium, which is a highly alkaline substance that interferes with the stomach acids. However, I was fortunate to not have gone through this symptom. One may experience loose bowls the first couple days and the reason is because the body is getting rid of the dead cancer cells and/or it might be a result from the required large doses of Vitamin C.

So far, every fact I have stated has been based upon my personal experience and knowledge. It's not meant to convey any impression or to try to convince others they will get the same results. My High pH Therapy consisted of 2 grams (a total of 6 grams of Cesium Chloride daily) 3 times a day, and Vitamins C, Vitamin A, Co-Q10, also Zinc, Selenium, and Potassium were also a part of my daily protocol.

Please note, it is very important that the Cesium and Potassium are not taken at the same time; take them an hour apart. This is to prevent cramping. If cramping occurs, however, increase the hour to two or three hours.

One day, I noticed a little dark blood in my urine. I was advised not to be alarmed that this was a good sign that the kidneys were doing their job.

How I Beat Cancer

Do your research as I did because there is a difference in the quality of Cesium Chloride and a dose for one brand may be dangerous or worthless compared to the same dose for another brand. The vendors, who are the experts in their specific products, should set the doses for each case.

As I mentioned earlier, always consult your health care professional to determine your dosage and what supplements you should use. Some doctors administer Nitrilosides in the form of laetrile (ingredient inside an apricot seed) because they believe it may be more effective than vitamins in enhancing the pickup Cesium by the cells.

One of the only downsides to this treatment is the potential for swelling and inflammation caused by the amount of cancer cells which are in the process of dying and the body's effort to get rid itself of the dead cells. I did not experience this side effect.

From my research, I discovered that there are times when a normal cell for some reason does not get a sufficient amount of oxygen. When this happens the problem may be that microbes have entered the cell, causing the cell to form a tuff protective cell membrane, which prevents oxygen from entering. When this takes place the oxygen level becomes too low and therefore to survive the cell becomes anaerobic. Being anaerobic they don't burn oxygen-they convert to ferment glucose to get its energy.

When there is no oxygen the glucose undergoes fermentation to create lactic acid. The lactic acid causes the cell's pH to drop from normal 7.3 down to 7 and lower to 6.5. In some cases it can drop as low as 5.7 which is an advance stage of cancer.

Because the cancer cells are burning glucose and creating lactic acid, a great deal of energy is being pulled from the non-cancerous cells. Once the lactic acid reaches the liver it is converted back to glucose. This is called the Cachexia Cycle and it continues while consuming large amounts of energy.

Chapter 3

Orthodox Treatments, Still No Cure

Dr. Hardin Jones, professor of medical physics at the University of California at Berkeley, has analyzed cancer survival statistics for 25 years. In 1969, at an American Cancer Society (ACS) meeting, he said, "Untreated patients do not die sooner than patients receiving orthodox treatment and in many cases they live longer." This assessment was subsequently supported by three other studies without any report of formal opposition.

According to Richard Walters, author of *Options: The Alternative Cancer Therapy Book*, groups of vested interlocking interests groups such as the ACS, National Cancer Institute (NCI), large pharmaceutical companies, insurance firms, hospitals, and medical schools preserve this status quo in cancer treatment and research. He asserted that this "medical cartel" is headed by the American Medical Association (AMA), "a trade union with an extremely powerful lobby." According to Walters, the AMA represents less than half the allopathic (conventional) doctors in the U.S. yet it has a stranglehold over government and American health care policies.

In 1987, the AMA was found guilty of restraint of trade in a "conspiracy to destroy and eliminate" the chiropractic profession, a legitimate competitor. Chiropractic physicians still have reporting requirements which allopathic physicians do not. The AMA continues to stage campaigns against alternative methods and doctors.

Today, in the U.S. and Canada, the powerful medical associations and cancer research organizations still shut down all competition, despite recent research showing therapies with cure rates higher than those obtained by chemotherapy and radiation. In fact, research has shown that in some cases conventional treatment is worse than no treatment at all yet surgery, chemotherapy and radiation continue to be the "treatments of choice."

In 1953, U.S. Justice Department lawyer, Benedict Fitzgerald, led an investigation into the cancer industry. He concluded that the AMA, NCI and FDA had entered into a conspiracy to promote surgery, radiation, and chemotherapy while suppressing promising therapies that were highly praised by patients who were cured. The government's response and solution to this issue-fire Fitzgerald.

Surgery

If surgery is the option you choose to cure your cancer there are a few things to think about. In the September 22, 1986 issue of *Business Week* it was noted that surgery, radiation, and chemotherapy all tend to fail for a very simple reason: A tumor the size of your thumb has one billion malignant cells in it. Even if a treatment gets 99.9% of them, a million remain to kill you. It also stated, "An operation on a bad malignant case is a very serious matter. Sometimes one gets a blaze up of toxemia. Further, cancer has very frequently spread far beyond the reach of operation and the operation shock hastens the spread of the virus and the death of the patient."

What about the myth of having lymph node surgery in an effort to remove every cancer cell. Patrick McGrady of *CANHELP* said, "Even though it's been proven conclusively that lymph node excision after radiation does not prevent the spread of cervical cancer, you will still see lymphadenectomices performed all over the country routinely." I knew a two women who had this procedure done and they both deeply expressed regret and claimed that they felt so bad they wish they were dead. It is a useless cure to the world of so-called medicine.

Radiation

It was Harvard University School of Public Health Professor, John Cairns, in 1985 who said that "the majority of cancers cannot be cured by radiation because the dose of x-rays required to kill all the cancer cells would also kill the patient." In 1980, Dr. Robert R. Jones said, "Many radiation complications do not occur for several years after treatment, giving the therapist and the patient a false sense of security for a year or two following therapy. The bone marrow, in which blood cells are made, is largely obliterated in the field of irradiation. This is an irreversible effect." In 1978, Dr. Lucien Israel, consultant to the NCI, said that people who undergo radiation therapy are more likely to have their cancer metastasize to other sites. Other studies have supported this view. He also stated that the "radioactivity intended to kill cancer cells can, instead, trigger mutations that create new cancer cells of other types."

According to several clinical trials and a study published in "The Lancet" a British medical journal, radiotherapy [radiation] following breast surgery increases death rates.

Dr. Irwin Bross, the former Director of Biostatistics at Roswell Park Memorial Institute, said in 1979, "For 30 years radiologists in this country have been engaged in massive malpractice." Needless to say that Bross was unable to get funding to research what he refers to as "doctor-caused cancer" from radiation therapy.

If these studies and quotes are true, why would a doctor continue to recommend radiation? They are fully aware of the side effects, which include severe, prolonged immune deficiency that could lead to other kinds of illnesses, and chromosomal damage, both of which can result in latter staged bouts with cancer. These are not "side effects" they are primary effects.

Radiation can cause nausea, vomiting, weakness, sores or ulcers, bone death following radiation of the mouth, welts and extensive burns of the skin, rectal ulcers, fistulas, bladder ulcers, colitis, swelling of a tumor after a large dose of radiation, which is especially dangerous for brain tumors, and severe fatigue where a patient could become bedridden. If these "side effects" were caused by an herbal treatment, a homeopathic one or any alternative treatment do you believe the treatment would be approved by the FDA and the AMA?

Dr. William Kelley, developer of an alternative, metabolic treatment said, "Often while making a biopsy the malignant tumor is cut across, which tends to spread or accelerate the [cancer] growth. Needle biopsies can accomplish the same tragic results. Surgery to remove the tumor can do the same thing." Dr. Kelley advises cancer patients to use homeopathic treatment to render the tumor harmless before attempting surgery, if surgery is the way you choose to go.

Chemotherapy

While waiting in the lobby of my doctor's office, I read in a medical journal magazine that the cancers most people die from like breast, colon, and lung generally do not respond to chemotherapy. Chemotherapy has only a limited effectiveness against any tumor that is large or has spread and the successes are generally with small, very early tumors. Several studies indicated that chemotherapy has no survival value in breast cancer.

In 1987, Dr. Alan Levin, Professor of Immunology, University of California Medical School said, "Most cancer patients in this country die of chemotherapy. Chemotherapy does not eliminate breast, colon or lung cancers. The fact has been documented for over a decade. Women with breast cancer are likely to die faster with chemotherapy than without it."

Dr. Levin, at a national conference on medical abuses, said, "Practicing physicians are intimidated into using regimes which they know do not work. One of the most glaring examples is chemotherapy, which does not work for the majority of cancers. Despite the fact that most physicians agree that chemotherapy is largely ineffective, they are coerced into using it by special interests groups which have vested interest in the profits of the drug industry."

Dr. John Cairns, Harvard University Professor of Microbiology. said, "Chemotherapy at most prevents perhaps 2% or 3% of the cancer deaths each year." If you have been diagnosed with cancer, find out if your type will be hurt or helped by chemotherapy.

Dr. Ulrich Abel, PhD. of West Germany, did a comprehensive study on chemotherapy. In 1990 he wrote, "There is no evidence for the vast majority of cancers that treatment with these drugs exerts any positive influence on survival or quality of life in patients with advanced disease." He also stated that although chemotherapy does shrink tumors initially in many patients, unfortunately this did not prolong survival because the cancer usually returned, often more aggressively than initially.

Abel surveyed hundreds of cancer doctors worldwide and he discovered that many oncologists would not take chemotherapy if they had cancer. Publicity about Abel's research was completely suppressed in the United States.

In the meantime, chemotherapy continues, despite the fact that all chemotherapy drugs are toxic and many are themselves carcinogenic.

Before you agree to surgery, radiation, and chemotherapy contact some of the consumer groups listed to get a second opinion about the effectiveness of these choices for your specific kind of cancer.

Chapter 4

It's All About Money

As stated earlier, from the moment you complete your last orthodox treatment to rid your body of cancer, according to the latest medical statistics, within five years the survival rate is only 3%. After I was diagnosed with prostate cancer, I learned that the cancer industry consisted of the pharmaceutical companies, the American Medical Association (AMA), American Cancer Society (ACS), the National Cancer Institute (NCI), and the Food and Drug Administration (FDA). It is my opinion that they are all responsible for 97% of the lives that have been lost to cancer. These industries are money driven; they treat the symptom and not the cause.

I often wondered why a company would even bother to research treatment for the symptoms of a disease. I then concluded that as long as they were treating the symptoms they don't have to cure the disease and therefore can continue writing prescriptions. The pharmaceutical companies are not interested in conducting studies to find a cure. Their only interest is making money. In 2014, a census reported that Americans spent twice as much on pharmaceuticals than any other country.

The following chart is an example of the profit-after mark-up-pharmaceutical companies are making from consumers of prescription medicine:

Product Name	Consumer Price	Cost of Ingredient	Mark Up
Prozac 20 mg	(100 tablets): $247.47	$0.11	224.973%
Tenormin 50 mg	(100 tablets): $104.47	$.013	80.362%
Prevacid 30 mg	(100 tablets): $ 44.77	$1.01	34,136%
Prilosec 20 mg	(100 tablets): $360.97	$0.52	69,471%
Celebrex 100mg	(100 tablets): $130.27	$0.60	21,712%
Claritin 10 mg	(100 tablets): $215.17	$0.71	30,306%
Norvasc 10 mg	(100 tablets): $188.29	$0.14	134,493%
Xanas 1 mg	(100 tablets): $136.79	$0.24	569,958%

I can't imagine how it is legal for big companies to take advantage of people who are in no position physically or financially to fight back. We elect officials to allow this to happen so I guess the government feels we are partially to blame. We need to hold officials accountable for this lack of protection. Maybe if we recall a few of them the seriousness of healthcare in America would take a front seat instead of sitting on the counter in a public restroom. Vote them out of office and choose leaders who will serve their constituents and not themselves. A mark-up by pharmaceutical companies is designed to cover other costs such as lobbyists, financing political campaigns, and television advertising. Again, it's all about money.

Have you ever noticed how a television commercial about a newly released "pill" on the market gives little information on the drug but an enormous amount on the side effects which could lead to suicide or death. How unbelievable that is to assume we are careless enough to overlook these facts. This explains why pharmaceutical companies "hire" politicians to fight their cause and hopefully keep us in the dark about alternative treatments.

With the gift of large donations, pharmaceutical companies have blocked the teaching of alternative cancer treatment in some medical schools around the country. They use the mass media and their money to disseminate false information discrediting alternative treatments and they use terms like "unproven treatments." The FDA and NIH control research money for alternative cancer treatments on live patients. They use congress to block any investigation of corruption in medicine and the ability to manufacture and distribute natural products by getting the FDA and FTC to not use the term "scientific evidence." In other words, pharmaceutical companies spend billions of dollars to keep alternative natural products and therapies from becoming known to the public.

Eventually the American people will wake up and demand answers to the questions that have plagued the progress of their health for decades. If we can go to the moon, invent electric cars, and cure Polio, why can't we find a cure for cancer?

There are more than 100 alternative treatments that are known to cure cancer. The best alternative method is a combination of several treatments and have been known to cure over 90% of those who have used them.

After over several years of research, I found that if pharmaceutical companies, our government, and the cancer associations would put their efforts behind alternative treatments they could save the lives of 99.9% of cancer patients. There is a cure, which I am not afraid to admit. Having cancer and healing from it should be no more serious than getting rid of a bad cold or Influenza.

What Is Cancer?

It never ceases to amaze me the surprising remarks I receive from the audience during my presentation on *How I Beat Cancer*. They have no clue about what cancer really is and they are convinced that once you are diagnosed with the disease, "it's the end." When I begin to explain how cancer can be cured with the proper treatment, the room become silent.

According to learned individuals, cancer is a disease in which healthy cells stop functioning and maturing properly. As the normal cycle of cell creation and death is interrupted these newly "mutated" cancer cells begin multiplying uncontrollably, no longer operating as an integrated and harmonious part of the body. They can also become parasitic and develop their own network of blood vessels to siphon nourishment away from the body's blood supply. This process, if unchecked, will eventually lead to the formation of a cancerous tumor. As the abnormal cells circulate within the bloodstream, the cancer can also spread to other parts of the body. This can cause the formation of more tumors and further sap the body's energy supply, weakening and eventually poisoning the patient with toxic byproducts.

Since 1890, doctors have theorized that fungal infections caused or contributed to the development of cancer. Fungus in the body will play havoc on our immune system and these fungi excrete toxins will continue to weaken and harm the body.

A particular fungus called Candida eliminate their waste which is acetaldehyde. This produces ethanol in the body. The results of the ethanol cause excessive fatigue and reduce strength and stamina. It also destroys enzymes that are needed for cell energy and inhibits the absorption of iron by the cells and causes damage to our DNA. Iron is one of the most important oxygen supports in the blood but the ethanol reduces the oxygen levels to the cells.

It has been proven that fungi is one of the causes of cancer. Some believe that cancer is a chronic infectious, fungus disease because fungal spores have been found in every sample of cancer tissue studied.

Alan Cantwell MD, the author of *Bacteria, the Ultimate Cause of Cancer* said, "If cancer is caused by infection or not, once the cancer cells get to the place where it is weakening the immune system the battle is on."

When the immune system has been compromised and the patient gets sick from one of the viruses, bacteria or fungi which have been in our body, creates a sickness. Our pH changes, hydration levels and cell voltage change, and all of these give way for the pathogens to move into our bloodstreams and tissues.

Cancer cells are always being created in the body. It is an ongoing process but the immune system-if healthy-is designed to find cancer cells and destroy them. The explosion of toxins and pollutants we are exposed to, junk foods we consume that are full of pesticides, mineral depleted soil that our foods are grown in, and cattle that are injected with growth hormones all contribute to weakening of our immune system. The internal environment of the body is prey to the over growth of cancer cells.

But don't be frightened, if you take care of your health and take action, you can change the internal environment to foster a healthy body that will attack cancerous cells and tumors by exploiting their weaknesses. Tumors are grown when more cancerous cells are created than the immune system can destroy.

All cancer begins in cells, the body's basic unit of life and it's helpful to know what happens when normal cells become cancer cells. A through explanation was once stated by the National Cancer Institute. "The body is made up of many types of cells. These cells grow and divide in a controlled way to produce more cells as they are needed to keep the body healthy. When cells become old or damaged, they die and are replaced with new cells. However, sometimes this orderly process goes wrong. The genetic material (DNA) of the cell can become damaged or changed, producing mutations that affect normal cell growth and division. When this happens, cells do not die when they should and new cells form when the body does not need them."

Wherever there is a proliferation of damaged cells, with walls that have changed and where oxygen cannot enter, when free radicals are in abundance and toxins are building up, when the mitochondria lose its ability to produce energy (ATP), when the cells pH becomes strongly acidic and cannot pull in necessary nutrients, the cell will rapidly change into a cancerous condition.

The body may form a mass of tissue called a tumor, but not all tumors are cancerous; tumors can be benign or malignant.

- Benign tumors aren't cancerous. They can often be removed, and in most cases, they do not come back. Cells in benign tumors do not spread to other parts of the body.
- Malignant tumors are cancerous. Cells in these tumors can invade nearby tissues and spread to other parts of the body. The spread of cancer from one part of the body to another is called metastasis.

Cancer is not just one disease but many and there are more than 100 different types. Most cancers are named for the organ or type of cell in which they start. For example, cancer that begins in the colon is called colon cancer, and the one that begins in the melanocytes of the skin is called melanoma.

Cancer types can be grouped into broader categories which includes:

- Sarcoma – cancer that begins in bone, cartilage, fat, muscle, blood vessels, or other connective or supportive tissue;
- Leukemia – cancer that starts in blood-forming tissue such as the marrow and causes large numbers of abnormal blood cells to be produced and enter the blood;
- Lymphoma and myeloma – cancers that begin in the cells of the immune system;
- Central nervous system cancer – cancer that begin in the tissues of the brain and spinal cord; and
- Carcinoma – cancer that begins in the skin or in tissues that line or cover internal organs. There are a number of subtypes of carcinoma, including adenocarcinoma, basal cell carcinoma, squamous cell carcinoma, and transitional cell carcinoma.

Rise In Statistics

According to the American Cancer Society and their 2014 annual report, that there will be an estimated 1,665,540 new cancer cases and 585,720 deaths steamed from the disease in the United States. Among men, prostate, lung, and colon cancer will account for about half of all newly diagnosed cases. Prostate cancer alone will account for about one in four cases. Among women, the three most common cancers in 2014 will be breast, lung, and colon, which together will account for half of all cases. Breast cancer alone is expected to account for 29% of all new cancers among women.

From 2006 to 2010, cancer incidence rates declined slightly in men by 0.6% per year and were stable in women, while the cancer death rate decreased by 1.8% per year in men and by 1.4% in women. The combined cancer death rate has declined for two decades. From a peak of 215.1 per 100,000 in 1991 to 171.8 per 100,000 in 2010 this 20 percent decline translates to the avoidance of approximately 1,340,400 cancer deaths (952,700 among men and 387,700 among women).

The magnitude of the decline in the cancer death rate from 1991 to 2010 varies substantially by age, race, and sex, with no decline among white women age 80 years and older to 55% decline among black men age 40 years to 49 years. Notably, black men experienced the largest drop within a 10-year age group.

To overcome cancer we must reverse the conditions that allow the cancer to develop and declare war on killing cancerous cells in our bodies.

Economic Impact

The financial costs of cancer are soaring every day. The expense is costly to the person with cancer and for society as a whole. The National Institute of Health (NIH) estimated that the 2009 total cost was $216.6 billion dollars. Direct medical costs (total of all health expenditures) was

$86.6 billion dollars.

These estimates are not comparable to those published in Cancer Facts & Figures before 2012. In 2011, the NIH began using a different data source: the Medical Expenditure Panel Survey (MEPS) of the Agency for Healthcare Research and Quality. The MEPS estimates are based on more current, nationally representative data and are used extensively in scientific publications. As a result, direct and indirect costs will no longer be projected to the current year, and estimates of indirect morbidity costs have been discontinued.

One of the major costs of cancer is the treatment, but the lack of health insurance and other barriers prevent many Americans from getting substantial basic health care. According to the U.S. Census Bureau, about 48.6 million people were uninsured in 2011 and about 10% of the children in the United States had no health insurance coverage in 2011. According to Cancer Facts & Figures, "Uninsured patients and those from ethnic minorities are substantially more likely to be diagnosed with cancer at a late stage, when treatment can be more extensive and more costly." This leads not only to higher medical costs, but also poorer outcomes and higher cancer death rates.

This year, about 585,720 U.S. residents are expected to die of cancer; that's more than 1,600 people a day. In the United States, cancer is the second most common cause of death exceeded only by heart disease and it accounts for about 1 out of 4 deaths.

The costs of treating cancer is billions of dollars. It empties our pockets and pierce our family's hearts. Reducing the barriers to eliminate suffering and to save lives is critical in this fight against cancer.

Chapter 5

The Misunderstanding

Much of the information in this chapter can be found in the report written by *Rev. Barbara Clearbridge, Entitled: Effective Non-Toxic Treatments for Cancer Are Available – If You Leave North America.*

Dr. Hardin Jones, Professor of medical physics at the University of California at Berkeley, analyzed cancer survival statistics for 25 years. In 1969, at an American Cancer Society (ACS) meeting, he said : "Untreated patients do not die sooner than patients receiving orthodox treatment, and in many cases they live longer." This negative assessment was subsequently supported by three other studies done by other researchers. No study has ever refuted these findings.

A group of vested, interlocking interests preserve the status quo in cancer treatment and research. This group includes the ACS, National Cancer Institute (NCI) National Cancer Institute, large pharmaceutical companies, and some insurance firms, hospitals, and medical schools, according to Richard Walters, author of "Options: the Alternative Cancer Therapy Book." He asserts that this "medical cartel" is headed by the American Medical Association (AMA), "a trade union with an extremely powerful lobby." According to Walters, the AMA represents less than half the allopathic (conventional) doctors in the U.S., yet has a stranglehold over government and American health care policies.

In 1987, the AMA was found guilty of restraint of trade in a "conspiracy to destroy and eliminate" the chiropractic profession, a legitimate competitor. Chiropractic physicians still have reporting requirements which allopathic physicians do not. The AMA continues to stage campaigns against alternative methods and doctors. This practice continues.

Today, in the U.S. and Canada, the powerful medical associations and cancer research organizations still shut down all competition, despite recent research showing therapies with cure rates higher than those obtained by chemotherapy and radiation. In fact, research has shown that in some cases conventional treatment is worse than no treatment at all. Yet surgery, chemotherapy and radiation persist as "treatment of choice."

In 1953, U.S. Justice Department lawyer Benedict Fitzgerald led an investigation into the cancer industry. The investigation concluded that the AMA, NCI and FDA had entered into a conspiracy to promote radiation, chemotherapy and surgery, while suppressing promising therapies that were highly praise by the cured patients themselves. What was the government's response? Fitzgerald was fired.

From Normal To Cancerous

I am often asked, "How does a normal cell become cancerous?" I explain to them that a normal cell does not turn cancerous in a short period of time. For some reason it first becomes mutated after being overtaken by microbes and damaged genes that control cell growth, division and its life span. One of the first things that happens is the cells begin to grow and multiply out of control. The mutated cell develops a hard membrane surface, and develops its own blood supply and begins to spread into other parts of the body via the bloodstream.

Normal cells usually stay in one place in your organ, and do not grow and multiply. For some reason if a normal cell of an organ become detached they self-destruct by a process known as apoptosis. With the cancer cell, the self-destruct does not happen, the cancer cell can grow and multiply without being attached to an organ. This allows them to enter the bloodstream and spread throughout the body.

In 1984, Keith Brewer, PhD (Physics) and H.E. Satori successfully treated thirty patients with various forms of cancer using Cesium Chloride, aka natures most alkaline mineral. All thirty patients survived.

They discovered that potassium, rubidium and Cesium are able to penetrate the membrane of the cancer cell surface. Glucose can still enter the cell but oxygen cannot. The cell then becomes anaerobic (able to live in the absence of oxygen). In the absence of oxygen, the glucose will ferment and cause lactic acid. The cell will drop to a low 6.5 at which Cesium rubidium and potassium can penetrate the cancer cell membrane raising the pH value to normal or it will eventually die.

The cancer cell taking into itself the Cesium and/or rubidium is the High pH therapy. This consists of the patient taking close to 6 grams of Cesium Chloride (2 grams, 3 times per day) an amount that should be sufficient to raise the pH in the cancer cells and bring them up in a few days to the pH level of 8 or above where a cancer cell cannot survive. At the same time, the presence of the Cesium and/or rubidium in the body fluids neutralizes the acid toxins leaking out of a tumor mass one may have rendering it nontoxic.

If you elect to try the High pH Therapy plan, make sure you consult your health care professional. Find a physician that will respect your decision to try an alternative treatment. If he or she does not, find one that will. It's your life on the line and it should be your decision. However, it is necessary to be monitored because your potassium, and magnesium levels must give a normal read.

Diet is very important. The basic diet during High pH Therapy is steamed or raw vegetables, and lots of fresh fruit. Some fruits such as oranges, which you may think to be acidic, are okay, because it will actually be processed by the body as alkaline.

Reduce the meats, especially red meats. You can eat fish or chicken at one of your meals a day. Be sure to drink plenty of water each day, eight to ten glasses.

High pH Therapy is the protocol I chose and followed when I was diagnosed with prostate cancer. I was informed that Cesium Chloride should always be taken with food. The first three days I opened the capsules and mixed the Cesium from the capsules with orange juice. It's not the best tasting stuff, but I soon got over it.

High pH Therapy Diet

The following was my diet and how I took the High pH Therapy:

Breakfast:

I took one gram Cesium Chloride (two capsules) in the morning with breakfast, and the following supplements: Zinc, Vitamin C (1000mg) Co-Q10 (200mg), and Potassium capsule daily (99 mg Magnesium).

Lunch:
Vegetables, raw or steamed and fruit with Vitamin C (1000mg), Potassium (99mg). I consumed as much fruit and vegetables that I desired.

Supper:
I took one gram (two capsules) Cesium Chloride, with my meal plus Vitamin C (1000mg), Magnesium (99mg).

Bedtime:
Eat a sandwich and a piece of fruit, one gram Cesium Chloride (two capsules) and Vitamin C (1000 mg), Potassium (99mg).

Eat as much fruit and vegetables as you wish, the more the better. During the protocol, I did experience some minor flu like symptoms, tingling sensations around the nose and lips and loose bowels. After the thirty days protocol, my PSA dropped from 3.7 to 2.01.

Due to the fact that your potassium levels will drop during this therapy, we are suggesting that before starting on the High pH Therapy you make arrangements with your physician to monitor your potassium levels, and prescribe the amount of potassium you should take. Check with your High pH therapy distributor, who may be able to refer you to a physician in your area.

I am often asked that if Cesium Chloride is such a "killer" of bad cancer then why haven't I heard of Cesium as a cancer therapy? The answer at its most fundamental level is money.

After using the High pH Therapy and spending less than $300.00, my personal opinion is that the Food and Drug

Administration, National Institution of Health, the CDC, and Medical societies like the American Medical Association , the Multinational Pharmaceutical Industries, and multi-billion dollar charitable institutions like the American Cancer Society, just to name a few, are interested in maintaining their power, prestige, and economics than they are in protecting the lives of myself and the millions of cancer patients diagnosed annually. It takes a great deal of time for new ways to fight cancer to be accepted.

Can you imagine if tomorrow these alternative methods were recognized and the old orthodox treatments were stopped, the billion dollar cancer industry would be out of business. They go to lengths to discredit and deny any natural treatment that will destroy a cancer cell and leave a normal cell intact.

For example, the medical establishment is interested in scientific evidence to support therapeutic claims. Yet, when the proof concerning Cesium is presented it is ignored. The evidence was presented in a series of double blind studies in 1980 by several institutions, which are known as the "Gold Standard." These tests demonstrate the ability of Cesium to target and kill cancer cells in a variety of tumors and to make it possible to determine the appropriate level of therapeutic in humans.

Dr. Keith Brewer Ph.d, physicist and former Director of the National Bureau of Standards Mass Spectroscopy Laboratory, conducted the first human tests of Cesium on terminal cancer patients. The results of the study stated that mass spectrographic and isotope studies have shown that potassium, rubidium, and especially Cesium are most efficiently taken up by cancer cells. This uptake was enhanced by Vitamins A and C as well as salts of zinc and Selenium. The quantity of Cesium taken up was sufficient to raise the cell to the 8 pH range.

This process occurs where cell mitosis creases and the life of the cell is short. Tests on mice fed Cesium and rubidium showed marked shrinkage in the tumor mass within 2 weeks. In addition, the mice showed none of the side effects of cancer. Tests have been carried out on over 30 humans. In each case the tumor mass disappeared.

All pain and effects associated with cancer disappeared within 12 to 36 hours; the more chemotherapy and morphine the patient received the longer the withdrawal period. Studies of food intake in areas were the incidences of cancer were very low showed that it met the requirements for the high pH therapy. As you may recall, these were terminal patients who exhausted all options and had doctors who concluded that the odds of living was stacked heavily against them.

Even so, the tumors were reduced in 30 out of 30 patients. This was a one hundred percent success rate with the benefit of not having any more pain associated with the tumor. Compare this with the twenty-five percent success rate of orthodox medicine. This was the "Phase II trial and the third element of the "Gold Standard," exactly the kind of scientific proof the medical establishment insists that is the only solution. When Dr. Brewer published his findings he was 90 years old and died two years later, making it impossible for him to defend his discovery.

Dr. H. Sartori MD completed two successful Phase II clinical trials and all that remained was the final step to start Phase III trials, which would have included thousands of patients and many institutions. But, the tragic outcome was Dr. Sartori was arrested and imprisoned on Rider's Island for ten months. During these ten months he was never charged and copies of Dr Brewer's papers were difficult to find.

The reason government sponsored clinical trials have not been conducted is that Cesium is a naturally occurring mineral and cannot be patented. The multinational Pharmaceutical Industry therefore can't make money, so research is discouraged.

Doctors are controlled by an industry that is making billions of dollars off expensive cancer fighting drugs and treatments. Medicine is an industry that does not look kindly on natural inexpensive supplements or alternative cancer treatments that cannot be patent. Natural substances may deprive "Big Pharma" of making outrageous profits on our suffering. It appears that most doctors promote and prescribe medications they are taught in medical school or introduced by a Big Pharma salesperson. Years from now, when we look back at conventional cancer treatments used by doctors, we will wonder why doctors prescribed chemotherapy and other orthodox treatments that damaged good cells and weakened our immune system that caused death.

One hundred years ago, we wondered why doctors would bleed a patient suffering from a disease that could have been cured by a home remedy or the use of leeches. I don't want to completely disregard orthodox treatments. I discovered that some have required that chemo be used with a non-orthodox product.

There is a treatment called "Insulin Potentiation Therapy" (IPT). This is a therapy where insulin is followed by a small dose of chemotherapy. The theory behind this is that cancer cells have fifteen times more insulin receptors than a normal cell. The insulin directs the chemo into the cancer cell because they have so many more insulin receptors, causing little damage to normal cells. It's documented that this therapy is about 80% effective when used with stage 1 and stage 2 cancers. With stage 3 and 4 cancers mixed results are reported. Yet even after twenty years of use, very few doctors use this therapy.

Oncologists make an inordinate amount of their income on chemotherapy drugs and radiation. To introduce this alternative treatment would only cost the patient between two to three hundred dollars.

Chapter 6

An Alkaline Body

It's very important to understand that there is a great difference in opinion to what constitutes a safe alkaline level for the blood and the body. The pH levels throughout our bodies do not react the same. For example, orthodox medicine determined that 8.0 or higher is considered to be fatal. However, my saliva test showed that I was at 8.0 for over a month during the time I was on the pH Therapy and according to my doctor I was healthy.

Orthodox medicine has been known to stretch the truth in order to discourage people from using alternative methods that have been proven to work. As I have stated numerous time throughout this book, I am not a physician, and I suggest you talk with your health care professional before making any decisions.

Saliva pH Test

This is a simple test you can conduct to measure your susceptibility to cancer, heart disease, osteoporosis, arthritis, and other degenerative diseases. In order to test your saliva or urine, you need to purchase pH strips at a drug store, health food store, or online. Whichever brand you buy, make sure that the range is appropriate.

For both urine and saliva tests, a pH range from 4.5 to 9.0 will give the best results. It is important to note that one reading is not enough to make any conclusions because your pH can be influenced by factors like what we eat and drink, stress, physical activity medications and nutritional supplements.

Saliva & Urine Test

Wait at least 2 hours after eating. Fill your mouth with saliva and then swallow. Repeat this step to make sure with the form of saliva you used in the first step. Then place the saliva onto pH paper and if it turns blue this indicates that the alkaline of your saliva is 7.4, which is a healthy pH. If the results are a different color, the chart will indicate the pH level. If your saliva is acidic (below the pH of 7.0) wait two hours and repeat the test.

While you sleep, your body is processing all the acids from the day. Therefore, it is advisable to take the test with the second urine of the day. The results are more reliable.

To take the urine test, pass the pH strip directly through your stream of urine. Wait about 15 seconds. Compare the color of the strip with the chart that comes with the pH strips. This is very easy and quick.

Saliva pH & Cancer

When healthy, the pH of blood is 7.4, the pH of spinal fluid is 7.4, and the pH of saliva is 7.4. Thus the pH of saliva parallels the extra cellular fluid pH test of saliva represents the most consistent and most definitive physical sign of the ionic calcium deficiency syndrome.

The pH of the non-deficient and healthy person is the 7.5 (dark blue) to 7.1 (blue) slightly alkaline range. The range from 6.5 (blue-green) which is weakly acidic to 4.5 (light-yellow) which is strongly acidic represents states from mildly deficient to strongly deficient, respectively. Most children are dark blue, a pH of 7.5. Over half of adults are green-yellow, a pH of 6.5 or lower, reflecting the calcium deficiency of aging and lifestyle defects. Cancer patients are usually a bright yellow, a pH of 4.5 especially when terminal.

Virtually all-degenerative diseases including cancer heart disease, arthritis, osteoporosis, kidney and gallstones, and tooth decay are associated with excess acidity in the body. While the body has a homeostatic mechanism that maintains a constant pH 7.4 in the blood, this mechanism works by depositing and withdrawing acid and alkaline minerals from other locations including the bones, soft tissues, body fluids and saliva. Therefore, the pH of these other issues can fluctuate greatly. The pH of saliva offers a window through which you can see the overall pH balance in your body.

Cancer cannot exist in an alkaline environment. All forms of arthritis are associated with excess acidity. Acid in the body dissolves both teeth and bones. Whatever health situation you are faced with, you can monitor your progress toward a proper acid alkaline balance by testing your saliva's pH.

Water (H_2O) ionizes into hydrogen (H+) and hydroxyl (OH-) ions. When these ions are in equal proportions, the pH is a neutral 7. When there are more (H+) ions than (OH-) ions then the water is said to be acid. If (OH-) ions outnumber the (H+) ions then the water is alkaline. The pH scale goes from 0 to 14 and is logarithmic, which means that each step is ten times the previous. In other words, a pH of 4.5 is 10 times more acid than 5.5, 100 times more acid than 6.5 and 1000 times more acid than 7.5.

Minerals & Food

Minerals with a negative electronic charge are attracted to the (H+) ions. These are called acid minerals. Acid minerals include: chlorine (CL-), sulfur (S), phosphorous (P-) and they form hydrochloric acid (HCl), sulfuric acid (H2SO4), and phosphoric acid (H3PO4). Minerals with a positive electrical charge are attracted to the negatively charged OH-ion. These are called alkaline minerals. Nutritionally important alkaline minerals include calcium (Ca+), potassium (K+), magnesium (Mg+), and sodium (Na+). Cancer patients tend to have an excess of sodium.

Also important for cancer treatment and prevention are the alkaline trace minerals rubidium and Cesium. To determine if a food is acid or alkaline, it is burned and the ash mixed with water. If the solution is acid or alkaline then the food is called acid or alkaline. Ash is the mineral content of food.

Why pH is Critical

Each cell in our body determines the overall health. If you have cancer or any other disease, the origin of that disease is at the cellular level not at the organ or system level. If your cell is healthy, your tissues are healthy, which creates healthy tissue, organs, and an immune system. All this combined play the part in creating a healthy body.

If the cell determines a healthy body, what constitutes a healthy cell? It is what we eat, drink, and breath. These components nourishes a cell with oxygen, water, vitamins, minerals, glucose, and amino acids, which is deposited in the bloodstream and flows to all the cells to nourish and remove acidic waste residues.

Our cells are a phenomenal within themselves, they are multifaceted constantly communicating like a wireless network with one another, controlling pH balance, temperature control, waste disposal, normal metabolized acids from body tissues and maintain health and vitality. All of this going on daily and while we are sleeping.

The pH of our tissues and body fluids affect the state of our health. The closer our pH is to 7.35 to 7.45 the higher our level of health and the more resistant we are to disease. It is the metabolic process that controls the pH of our body.

When the acids begin to build up in our body's cells are poisoned and start to corrode, then tissue corrode, slowly corroding our veins and arteries, which is what is called hemorrhage. If left unchecked all cellular activities and functions will cease leading to death. The medical community refers to this as a degenerative disease.

On a daily basis our body struggles to manifesting severe imbalances. All of our metabolic processes which include our immune system depend on a delicately balanced pH which works in balance with our electromagnetic energies. Also very importantly the body fights to maintain the blood pH at 7.35-7.45 and our temperature of 98.6 degrees.

Dr Gary Tunsky in his article "pH of the Human Body is Critical for health." He talks about "seven homeostatic adaption responses that fight to maintain this pH balance."

(1) Using high pH body fluids such as water as a solvent by neutralizing acid residues

(2) Pulling bicarbonate from the pancreas into the blood (an alkalizing agent). Bicarbonate ions are generated into the blood cells from carbon dioxide and diffuse into the plasma.

(3) Protein buffers of glutathione, methionine, cystine, taurine, just to name a few, act as buffers intra-cellularly to bind or neutralize acids during cellular disorganization.

(4) Electrolyte buffers of sodium, calcium and potassium work in the blood, lymph, and extra cellular and intracellular fluids to bind acids, which are then removed through the urine.

(5) Pulling stored calcium and magnesium from skeletal bones and teeth to neutralize blood acids.

(6) Filtration and elimination of acidic residues through the skin, urinary tract and respiration.

(7) Pushing blood acid residues and accumulated toxins into outer extremities as a storage bin away from vital organs. The wrist, joints, fingers, toes and skin are the major target areas to keep the toxins from saturating internal vital organs like the heart and lungs.

When all seven protected phases are overwhelmed, the end result is accumulated, acid residues at the cellular level, which drown out oxygen. The final result is death. Dr. Tunsky's original titled was called, "What In The Cell Is Going On?: The battle is over pH."

Chapter 7

Amygdalin

In spite of the great advances in the diagnosis and treatment of malignant tumors, cancer continues to be one of the leading causes of death in the United States. It has been stated by the American Cancer Institute that "one out every four persons die of cancer." Cancer is the number two killer following heart attacks. It is true that the old orthodox methods of treatment; chemotherapy, surgery, and radiation, are capable of curing some patients but, the mortality rate has not improved substantially in the past 25 years. Almost sixty percent of the patients, upon being diagnosed find that their disease is so widespread that the chemotherapy drugs currently being used, cannot be given in dosages sufficient to destroy the large tumor, because of the high toxicity of the drug. Because of the adverse effects of chemotherapy and other cancer drugs, many cannot undergo surgery or radiotherapy.

Because of these problems it is imperative that we look to other methods of treatment or alternative treatments that have little or no toxicity in therapeutic doses. In the last fifteen years, many vegetable and hormonal substances have been discovered that has been proven to attack and destroy cancer cells in the body and have no effect on the normal cells. One of these vegetable agents, whose anti-tumor actions has been known for many years and has been scientifically proven, yet FDA and large pharmaceutical companies has fought against an anti-tumor agent know as AMYGDALIN or commonly known as Laetrille).

Laetrile is the trade name for laevo-mandelonitrile-beta-glucuronoside. This product was synthesized by Ernst T. Krebs Jr. which was originally patented to treat "disorders of intestinal fermentation." This compound has similar molecules related to amygdalin.

Amygdalin was isolated among other enzymes as far back as 1830 by two French chemists. They found that amygdalin contained two molecules of glucose one molecule of hydrogen cyanide and on molecule of benzaldhyde.

Even though cyanide is poisonous, in this combination it is not poisonous in the body; "the normal cells contain an enzyme called Rodhenase which "neutralizes" the laetarile.. This enzyme does not allow laetrile to release the cyanide. Therefore, laetrile only serves as glucose to healthy cells providing energy. The cancerous cells do not contain this enzyme. In the absence of Rodhenase, the laetrile is activated liberating the cyanide radical inside the cancerous cell causing its destruction, but has no effect on the normal cells."

As the cancer cells are attacked by the laetrile it transforms into silicate which is similar to aspirin, contributing to pain control.

There are some limitations when using laetrile to treat cancer; it is more effective in the most common tumors such as Carcinoma of the Lung, Breast, Prostate, Colon and Lymphomas.

Laetrile is a natural chemotherapeutic substance that can be found in a variety of vegetables and seeds. The greatest concentration can be found in the seeds of the rosaceous fruits, such as apricot pits, peach pits, and other bitter nuts.

How I Beat Cancer

In 1981, the National Cancer Institute (NCI) conducted clinical trials that were highly publicized, and tried unsuccessfully to prove that laetrile was ineffective and toxic. However, today laetrile is known as one of the successful alternative cancer therapies. Laetrile has been found to be effective on patients that have an active cancer, and effective with maintenance of remission, and prevention of cancer. It has also been proven that laetrile's non-toxicity permits its use indefinitely in the prevention of relapses and the prevention of the spread of the cancer to other parts of the body.

Cancer is prevalent in all age levels in all lifestyles, and it appears that cancer is a man-made disease and therefore a preventable disease. Cancer is caused through our diets; food additive, pesticides, ultraviolet radiation and a variety of other environmental factors are directly implicated.

If we look at history as far back as the building of the pyramids, or China before the mention of Christ, documents mention the therapeutic use of derivatives of bitter almonds.

I don't want to rule out the fact that the orthodox treatments don't help some people, but the death rate from cancer is increasing. Many patients cannot be exposed to chemotherapy, surgery or radiotherapy because of the undesirable effects over their poor physical condition results from cancer. And, these orthodox treatments are really destroying our immune systems that take away the odds of being cured. Actually only 3% of the patients using the orthodox methods of treatment survive. Shocking as it may be, this is the truth the cancer industry do not want you to know.

This being said, it's justified that the search for new substances with anti-tumor effects and with little or no toxicity be found.

Many Americans have been going to Mexico for treatment, because in the U.S. the Food and Drug Administration has used regulation, not laws, to keep doctors in some states from using Amygdalin (laetrile) therapy. There is no federal law against laetrile, nor does laetrile appear on any official list of prescribed items. The FDA has also used regulation, not law, to ban the interstate shipment and sale of laetrile by alleging that it is either an unlicensed new drug or an unsafe or adulterated food or food additive. It is neither.

Amygdalin is an extract of apricot kernels, which makes it a food supplement and nothing more. Vitamin B-17 was the subject of great controversy 25 years ago when some of the world's top scientists claimed that when consumed, its components make it 100% impossible for an individual to develop cancer and will kill existing cancer. "Pharmaceutical companies pounced on this claim immediately and demanded that FDA studies be conducted. Pharmaceutical companies conduct studies on patented chemicals they invent, so that at the end of their study, if the drug gets approved, they have exclusive rights to its sale. They never conduct studies on foods that cannot be patented and that can be sold at any supermarket as a supplement. Foods that contain Vitamin B-17 are: Kernels or seeds of fruit.

Kills Only Cancer Cells

It is very important to understand that several enzymes are found in our body that performs many different tasks. There is one enzyme called Rhodanese that is found in large quantities throughout the body, but not found where there are cancer cells. But where ever you find cancer you will find another enzyme called Beta-Glucosidase. Rhodanese is not found where there are cancer cells and Beta-Gluscosidase is found in large quantities where there are cancer cells.

When the B-17 comes into contact with cancer cells, there is no rhodanese to break it down and neutralize but instead, only the enzyme beta-gucosidase is present in very large quantities. When B-17 and Beta-Glucosidase come into contact with each other, a chemical reaction occurs and the Hydrogen Cyanide and Benzaldehyde combine to produce a poison that destroys and kills the cancer cell.

Amygdalin (laetrile) contains four substances. Two are glucose, the third is benzaldehyde, and the fourth is cyanide. Cyanide and benzaldehyde are poison if they appear as free molecules not bound within other molecular formations. Many foods, including vitamin B-17, contain cyanide. But they are safe because the cyanide remains bound and locked as part of another molecule. There is an enzyme in normal cells to catch some free cyanide molecules and render them harmless by combining them with sulfur. That enzyme is the rhodanese. By binding the cyanide to sulfuric rhodanese, it is converted to a cyanate, which is a neutral substance. It is then easily passed through the urine without causing harm to the normal cell.

Cancer cells thrive on fermenting sugar instead of metabolizing with oxygen. Amygdalin contains two glucose molecules so the amygdalin molecules are quite appealing to sugar hungry cancer cells. And cancer cells contain an enzyme that normal cells do not share-beta-glucosidase.

This enzyme is considered the unlocking enzyme for amygdalin molecules. It releases both the benzaldehyde and the cyanide, creating a toxic synergy that destroys cancer cells. The beta-blucosidase enzyme causes cancer cells to self destruct by opening themselves to the cyanide and benzaldehyde. This is how cancer cells are tricked and targeted by amygdalin. Chemotherapy does not discriminate. It kills healthy cells and destroys the immune system.

I know I mentioned this process earlier in the book but I feel it crucial to emphasize that laetrile is not a magic bullet. This is not the case and there are factors that we have to consider.

One is the type of cancer. Some types of cancer may respond to a treatment more readily than another. Laetrile is not equally effective on all types of cancers. Laetrile is more effective against adenocarcinoma, Hodgkin's disease and less effective on sarcomas and melanomas, and the results are poor results on leukemia. Research has shown that Laetrile Therapy has been successful with lung, prostate, breast, liver, lymphomas, and brain cancer. The chemical quality of laetrile, however, has a great deal to do with therapeutic results.

It's very important that high quality laetrile be used. If this point is not recognized, inadequate dose levels and false negative therapeutic results may occur. The amount of laetrile that is administered is a factor. In the past, most physicians have given a dosage that was too little. If adequate blood levels are to be maintained, the frequency and route of administration, and the dosage are very important.

The most effective administration of laetrile is by intravenous injection. Do not take the necessary dosage my mouth. A factor that should be kept in mind is the tissue damage caused by radiation and toxicity. The result from chemotherapy has a lot to do with patient recovery.

It has been noted that 90% of patients using laetrile used other types of cancer therapies that failed. It is the opinion of some metabolic physicians that if the patient had started laetrile therapy when they were diagnosed, they stand a better chance of the cancer going into remission.

Liver function is very important in cancer therapy. The liver has extremely complex metabolic functions. It stores essential vitamins, such as A, D, B-12, and iron in the form of ferritin. The liver also forms a large proportion of the blood constituents: Fibrinogen, Prothrombin, Accelerator globulin, Factor VII, and other coagulation factors. The liver also plays an effective part in the vascular storage and the filtration of blood, with about 1000ml of blood flowing through the liver portal vain and the sinusoids each minute with an additional 400 ml flowing into the sinusoid and the hepatic artery. So if the liver or kidneys are compromised by cancer there is an adverse affect to the entire metabolism of the body.

Studies conducted that the use of laetrile indicate there is no damage to the liver or interference with the function of the kidney. The reason for the great effort placed into the metabolic therapy is to sustain adequate liver and kidney function and to minimize the detoxification load placed upon these vital organs.

Laetrile Therapy is the most effective method when used in conjunction with a comprehensive metabolic approach and it is most effective when used with adequate nutritional support, mineral supplements, and vitamins. Patients are placed on a vegetarian diet which includes fresh fruits and vegetables and a reduction of proteins, refined sugars, fats, and processed foods.

It is necessary to have a detoxification protocol. The treatment requires for the patient to take a minimum of 9 grams of laetrile per day. The dose is administered by the intravenous route. Sometimes larger doses are given. If the patient refuses to follow the general Metabolic Program then the laetrile protocol is not recommended.

Due to political pressures on the FDA, within the next few years, laetrile will be legalized in the United States. However, it is unfortunate that until then people will suffer and die in the name of orthodox medicine (chemotherapy, radiation and surgery). The suppression of information on cancer treatments and cures are allowed only because it is a money maker for the pharmaceutical companies. It is an outright shame that our government allows this to exist, which is a flagrant violation of the antitrust laws of this country.

Have you ever noticed the amount of pharmaceutical ads on television? The media is just as guilty as the drug companies. Only a portion of the side effects are reported because the goal is to advertise the benefits so the consumer will purchase the drug.

The 14th amendment of the United States Constitution states:

NO STATE SHALL MAKE OR ENFORCE ANY LAW WHICH SHALL ABRIDGE THE PRIVILEGES OR IMMUNITIES OF THE CITIZENS OF THE UNITED STATES: NOR SHALL ANY STATE DEPRIVE ANY PERSON OF LIFE, LIBERTY, OR PROPERTY WITHOUT DUE PROCESS OF LAW, NOR DENY TO ANY PERSON WITHIN ITS JURDISDUCTION THE EQUAL PROTECTION OF THE LAW.

Dr. Ernest T. Krebs, a biochemist who discovered Vitamin B-17 at the beginning of 1950, said, "Seven apricot seeds per day will make it impossible to develop cancer." One or two vitamin B-17 tablets (100mg) are an acceptable supplemental dosage per day.

Hospitals in Mexico that use this protocol is Contreras Hospital and Del Reo Hospital in Tijuana. They claim a 100% recovery rate with patients who have not received chemo and/or radiation because of the amount of damage to the liver. The other hospital is Harold Manner. They have successfully treated over 100,000 cancer patients over the last thirty years.

Del Reo Hospital has a 21 day therapy in which they include the typhoid vaccine, the B-1 (9 grams per day), pancreatic enzymes, vitamin C, whole foods that contain B-17, and pancreatic enzymes (apricot seeds and pineapple juice). No other clinic or hospital in the world uses these powerful protocols-only parts of it.

Chapter 8

Miracle Mineral Supplement

While gathering research to write this book, I came across a gentleman who lives in my hometown of Nevada. He said he knew of a miracle mineral supplement (MMS) that would cure not only malaria, it's sole purpose, but also cancer, arthritis, hepatitis, herpes, aids, and other deadly diseases.

I was hesitant to continue reading about this so-called "miracle cure" because it seem too good to be true and I did not have time to waste. But then again what did I have to lose; the arthritis in my knees was getting worse and I was desperate for pain relief. Prior to discovering the benefits of MMS, I went to my primary care physician seeking some help for my arthritis and was referred to a Rheumatologist.

On my first visit to the specialist, I had blood work done. Two weeks later, I went to my second appointment and was told my panel results were "positive." He said, "Your diabetes level is good, the red and white corpuscles are in order, but there is not much I can do about your arthritis so you just have to deal with the pain and discomfort for now."

I was shocked to hear such nonsense and my face resembled how I felt. He continued to stress his point. "After all Mr. Gaines you are in your seventies so be grateful that's the only problem you have to worry about." I said, "So are you saying that if I was 25 years old, you would have something to prescribe me?" I couldn't comprehend why a Rheumatologist would give such distasteful advice. He then said, "Just drink a couple bottles of Gatorade each day and before bedtime a glass of tonic water. This may help you."

I returned to my primary care physician and reported what I was told. He suggested a second opinion. After my first visit to this specialist, the advice was pretty much the same. He said, "There is not anything I could do except put you on some medication, and the meds may have some horrible side effects." I declined. Like I said what did I have to lose.

During my continued research on MMS, I stumbled across a book by Jim V. Humble, "Breakthrough: The Miracle Mineral Supplement of the 21st Century." It was written as a cure for malaria but I found the information to be quite helpful for understanding the body and the various levels of disease. Jim is so committed to healing people, he would mail a free copy to anyone who are experiencing hard financial times.

For the sake of the arthritis in my knees, I purchased a MMS kit for $28.00, a year supply, which included a 4oz bottle of MMS and a 4oz bottle of activator. You can mix it at home and the taste is tolerable.

Jim Humble claims in his book that normal arthritis is caused by muscles in an area that pull in the "wrong direction." When this happens, they create pain and begin to deteriorate the joint.

I ingested the MMS and rubbed DMSO (Dimethyl Sulfoxide) on my knees. After five days, the pain was 90% gone. I discontinued the DMSO and the only difference was a little stiffness in my knees when I stood up which subsided when I began to walk.

Multiple Ways Used

MMS is 28% Sodium Chlorite, and when mixed with vinegar or the activator, it generates chlorine dioxide (CLO_2). The reason why this happens is because the acetic acid in the vinegar causes the solution to be slightly acidic. The MMS is normally alkaline. When it is made acetic, by adding the vinegar, it becomes slightly unstable and it begins to release chlorine dioxide. When we add apple juice (or any non vitamin C juice) it dilutes the solution so that there is about 1 parts per million (ppm) of chlorine dioxide in the total apple juice mixture. Inside the stomach, the MMS generates chlorine dioxide, but at a slower rate, and continues to generate chlorine dioxide for the next 12 hours.

The red blood cells that normally carry oxygen throughout the body have no mechanism to differentiate between chlorine dioxide and oxygen. In the walls of the stomach, where the blood picks up nutrients of various kinds and when a chlorine dioxide ion touches a red blood cell, it is accepted.

If a cancer cell or a parasite is present, it will be destroyed as well as the chlorine dioxide. If there are no harmful parasites, cancer cells, or harmful particles in the body, the chlorine dioxide will be carried by the red blood cell to some point in the body where oxygen would normally be used to oxidize poisons and other harmful things. It is there the chlorine dioxide is released. The chlorine dioxide has over a hundred times more energy to do the same thing the oxygen does without hurting healthy cells because the immune system has the chlorine dioxide under control.

If the chlorine dioxide does not interrupt anything that can set it off, it will begin to deteriorate and gain an electron or two. This may allow it to combine with other substances to create a very important substance that the immune system utilizes to make hypochlorous acid.

Hypochlorous acid is probably the most important acid of the immune system. It kills pathogens, killer cells, even cancerous cells. When the body has a deficiency of this substance it is called myeloperoxidase deficiency. Many people are afflicted with this deficiency, which can increase during diseased levels, because the immune system needs a great deal of this acid to restore a healthy body.

Chlorine dioxide also tends to neutralize poisons. Almost all substances that are poisonous to the body are, to some extent, acetic in nature or below the neutrality of the body. The chlorine dioxide will neutralize many of these poisons. In his book, Jim Humble talks about a dog that was bitten by a rattlesnake. He was given a dose of MMS every half hour and within a few hours the dog was healed.

Protocol

Start with 2 to 6 drops of MMS in an empty glass; add 2 to 6 drops of 5% hydrochloric acid solution activator or lime or citric acid solution for each drop of MMS. Wait three minutes, add a half glass of water or apple juice then drink. (Use only a non vitamin "C" Juice). At the end of the day, repeat the same process but increase the drops by one. If you have a viral disease, increase the number of drops each hour or several times a day for diseases caused by bacteria or pathogens to 3, 4, 6 and to 15. Stay at 15 drops a day for several days and then increase to twice a day.

If you do not notice any improvements, increase the number of drops up to 20 or 25 drops, or even as much as 30 in small doses throughout the day. Reduce the number of drops if you feel nauseous, but start increasing them right away as best as you can.

Do not remain at 20 to 30 drops unless you really see an improvement in the condition you are trying to address. When the condition has been overcome, decrease to 6 drops a day for maintenance. Don't be alarmed if you experience nausea, vomiting, or diarrhea. It is simply the body's way to get rid of dead cells.

Chapter 9

Photon

The Photon Protocol is one of the most powerful of the protocols mentioned in this book. This protocol is for patients who have very dangerous tumors and a weak immune system from chemotherapy or radiation.

As I mentioned earlier, cancer is caused by a weak immune system. We all have cancer cells in our body but if we are fortunate enough to have a strong immune system, the immune system will destroy any cancer cell that attempts to grow. Otherwise, the number of cells can spiral out of control.

What causes the immune system to become weak? It starts with microbes and parasites in the organs. The glucose in the organ that the cells normally eat are eaten by the microbes and/or parasites which causes the normal cells to become weak mainly due to a lack of food. Our organs are made up of cells and without food the cells become weak.

The microbes and parasites excrete mycotoxins (waste) which are acidic and weakens the organs. It is necessary that the organs maintain a balance or they will cause the immune system to weaken and the cancer cells to proliferate.

The Photon Protocol can be used for almost any form of cancer, but is especially important with patients that have a microbe-oriented type of cancer, such as: melanoma, sarcomas, cervical cancer, ovarian cancer and uterine cancer. Photon Protocol is important if the patient has a dangerous tumor near the heart, inside the lungs, in the throat, in the brain, and if they are suffering from diabetes, or an infection.

What sets the Photon Protocol apart from some other protocols is that it address the "root cause" of the cancer. These treatments address the cellular energy issues as well as the microbial issues.

The Photon Protocol includes treatments that address the immune system and dangerous tumor microbes in the bloodstream and infections in other major organs such as the pancreas, liver, gallbladder, and cellular energy.

This protocol gives the patient added time to deal with the "root cause" of their weakened immune system. If you don't want the cancer to return, you must deal with the "root cause."

Cancer is an energy and a microbial disease. The two items are connected because microbes and their mycotoxins are what weaken the organs and cause cancer at the cellular level. Weak organs lead to a weak immune system and a weak immune system can create a safe-haven for microbes and cancer cells. It is important to note that the Photon device is considered to be only a partial treatment for cancer.

The first half of the treatment is a consultation with the Ed Skilling Institute. The consultation will entail a nutritional protocol; the results will lead to targeting particular microbes which are the cause for your weakening immune system. By following the nutritional protocol you will restore balance between the organs and restore the immune system. Once the immune system is functioning as intended, it will be able to fight off the cancer cells. The Photon is an electro-medicine device that energizes the cells and other positive affects in the body.

Testimonial

My name is Floyd Jackson, I am fortunate to have been using the Photon Genie for over five years now. I am 52 years old and in the last few years, I have been experiencing the most stable health ever; more than any time in m whole life. I'm grateful for these power tools and how they enhance the quality of my life and they keep on "giving." I continue to experience new levels of health.

Over time, these technologies dynamically promote more harmony and balance blood pressures, blood sugars, neurotransmitters, hormones, chemistries, and weight. The body is more able to make what it needs. The detoxification and light energies help the body to move and balance and alleviate blockages, resistances, obstructions, pain working at the cause level from the inside out. I now take a fraction of the supplements and get more benefit compared to five years ago. I digest better, sleep better, and both my heart and liver are stronger and healthier now.

On a scale of 1 to 10, the energy for my heart has gone from a level "5" to level "10" and my liver has gone from a level "4" to a level "9." I have learned first-hand that we underestimate the amount of infection the body is dealing with and what it takes to overcome all of it. Both the Photon Genie and the Photon Genius help the body overcome infections by providing energy and power to help the body heal renew, regenerate, revitalize. What a great blessing; I encourage everyone to experience as many sessions as possible. I plan on doing them the rest of my life. It is just too easy and the benefits are priceless!

Floyd Jackson,
Beaver Falls Pennsylvania

Electro-Medicine

Electro-medicine is a discipline within the field of medicine that uses electronics and energy technologies to aid in the treatment of a variety of physical symptoms, ailments and disease conditions.

In 1930, a gentleman by the name of Dr. Royal Rife invented the first microscope that was capable of viewing a live virus. It was the first microscope capable of 60,000 magnifications. A regular microscope cannot see a virus because the virus is smaller than the wavelength of light, and an electron microscope will kill the virus.

With the Rife microscope, he was able, for the first time, to see the virus or microbe within a cell. It was also believed at that time that these microbes were responsible for causing health problems and possibly cancer.

Rife was able to develop a method for killing these microbes by using electronic frequencies. He found that cells oscillate at certain frequencies and therefore was able to tune in on a particular cell that could destroy a microbe. It was also noted that this method could also destroy cancer cells.

Years later, following Dr. Rife's methods, Dr. Bob Beck, Dr. Hulda Clark, and Georges Lakhovsky researched and built machines that can eliminate viruses, parasites, fungi, bacteria and pathogens in our body using electrical currents and frequencies.

Dr. Bob Beck built the Blood Electrifier and the Magnetic Pulse Generator. He proved that by removing the viruses, parasites, fungi, bacteria and pathogens from the body, the immune system would strengthen effectively fight off cancer in the body.

Dr. Hulda Clark invented the "Zapper." The Zapper

works on the basis of electrical frequency. Her zapper is known to kill viruses, fungi and parasites as well as destroying cancer cells. It must be noted that if you are in advanced stages of cancer it is best to use a couple alternative treatments while also using the electronic medical devices. Using the zapper and the magnetic pulse generator takes time to destroy the microbes in the body before the immune system gets stronger.

The body naturally contains electricity and it controls the function of every cell. A variety of electrical impulses help facilitate bodily functions including actions needed for health maintenance, healing, and regeneration. By programming the cells of the body with the harmonic electrical impulses that occur in a perfect state of health, we can help trigger and redirect them.

Equally important, we have "electric-powered" energetic brains. Our thoughts and perceptions consist of complex networks of energetic fields and electrical signals that pulse and sweep throughout the brain and nervous system. So it makes sense that harmonic, electrical revitalization of the cells and functions of the brain can work to balance and improve your mental and emotional state as well as destroy unwanted pathogens. Electro-medicine helps the body build the immune system which controls and eliminates the cancer in the body.

As far back as 1859, individuals have been experimenting with electro-medicine to cure diseases. Nikola Tesla, in 1895, read his published article "High Frequency Oscillators for Electro-Therapeutic and Other Purposes" at the eighth annual meeting of the American Electro-Therapeutic Association in Buffalo, NY. He stated the harmlessness of passing great amounts of electrical energy throughout the body without causing pain or serious discomfort.

In an 1898 article, he concluded that the bodily tissues are condensers and the basic component (dielectric) for equivalent circuit was developed for the human body. He said the relative permittivity for tissue is at a very low frequency from 10 Hz to 100 Hz. Radio Frequency 10 kHz to 100 MHz exceeds most commercially available dielectrics on the market. He claims that our bodies have an inherent adaption to high voltage electronic field and this is due to high trans-membrane potential already present in our cellular tissue.

By September of 1932, at the American Congress of Physical Therapy in New York, Dr. Gustave Kolischer announced that Tesla's high-frequency electrical currents were showing great promise in destroying cancer cells in the body.

In 1922, a Russian doctor and histologist, Alexander Gurvich and his wife, discovered that living cells separated by quartz glass were able to communicate vital-cell information. It was suggested after many experiments that the information was transmitted by invisible light waves in a UV frequency spectrum passed by quartz and stopped by window glass.

Dr. Gurvich determined that muscle tissue, cornea, blood, and nerves are all transmitters of this special energy. His work is the first documented evidence of "biophotons", coherent light emitted by animal and plant cells, which later became the basis for the design of later bioelectro magnetic therapy devices.

In 1925, Georges Lakhovsky published a paper with the explicit title, "Curing Cancer with Ultra Radio Frequencies." He found that cell oscillations must reach a certain value before the organism is strong enough to repulse the destructive vibrations from certain microbes.

He also believed you should not kill the microbes in contrast with the healthy cells, but to reinforce the oscillations of the cell either directly by reinforcing the radio activity of the blood or producing on the cells a direct action by means of the proper rays.

Lashovsky's Radio-Cellulo-Oscillator (RCO) produced low frequency all the way through gigahertz radio waves with lots of extremely short harmonics. He favored such a wide bandwidth device so that "the cells with very weak vibrations, when placed in the field of multiple vibrations, finds its own frequency and starts again to oscillate normally through the phenomenon of resonance."

As a result, Lakhovsky's RCO is often called MWO (multiple wave oscillator) for these reasons. The MWO uses a Tesla coil and special antenna with concentric rings that induce multiple sparks between them.

In 1959, Ed Skilling was commissioned by several California cancer doctors to evaluate a $30,000 Rife instrument. His investigation determined that Rifle's frequency theory was not accurate and he took electro-medicine in a new direction, applying space age electronics. He said, "The only known cure for Cancer (or anything else) is your own god-given immune system."

Skilling became more committed to his research after several family members died from cancer. Using space age electronics, he concluded that the human body itself produces the great life restoring energy and chemistry needed for good health, and the Photon Genius and Photon Genie dynamically triggers this chemical and energetic balancing effect to promote the body to be the best it can be.

Another very important contribution to Electro-medicine was when Dr. Bob Beck discovered the idea of purifying the blood and destroying microbes in the blood.

This is done by placing two electrodes harmlessly on the skin, directly over the arteries, on the ankles or wrist and wired to an electronic device that is capable of painlessly injecting currents into the bloodstream through the skin.

A controlled amount of electrical current thus passes through the circulatory system while the patient rests or undertakes a quiet activity. Even though the electric current apparently does not kill all the viruses, research has shown that it deactivates all of them so that they lose the ability to infect cells. Viruses that can't penetrate cells are fair game for removal by the immune system. Therefore, during the period of treatment, the immune system can successfully remove these deactivated viruses from the body. Bacteria, fungus and parasites in the blood are also neutralized or killed by the electric current.

In 1980, Dr. Clark discovered the same principles as Dr. Beck. Through Dr. Clark's use of her Frequency Generator she called the "Digital Zapper", which was used primarily to research specific frequencies, she found that certain pathogens and parasites could be eliminated in the body.

Dr. Clark would dial up a frequency and record the point where the pathogen would literally explode through the electro-frequency impulses. She strongly suggested that it was best, if you can afford it, to buy the "Digital" type Zapper. The principles of the Zapping pathogens as specific frequencies are far more superior than a single frequency. Dr Clark also understood that her "Digital Type Zapper" powered by electricity not battery could provide a far greater power amperage. Her machine was not affected by problems associated with batteries; it could make use of frequencies up to 1 Million Hertz.

Immune System

The immune system is an immensely complicated and intricate combination of many systemic and bodily functions. It represents the totality of all of the complex and interrelated living processes. Your immune system is what enables you to resist attacks from diseases and overcome infections. It is the primary essential requirement for survival since we are surrounded by viruses, bacteria, parasites, and toxins. Elements of the immune system penetrate all of the tissues and organs of the body, vigilantly defending against every manner of threat.

The immune system integrates and manages all of the tissues and organs of the body with a kind of cellular intelligence in the form of exquisitely sophisticated electrical and chemical communication systems. This dazzling communications system, which manages and orchestrates all of our many defenses, extends throughout the entire body and involves every cell of our body.

The immune response has two general aspects: Nonspecific defenses include physical and chemical barriers. The inflammatory response and interferon's are the body's initial reaction to any kind of injury, whether it was due to trauma, a foreign organism, a chemical toxin, or localized oxygen deprivation. Physical barriers include the intact skin and mucous membranes. These barriers are aided by various antimicrobial chemicals in tissue and fluids. An example of such a substance is lysozme, an enzyme present in tears, that destroys the cell membranes of certain bacteria.

The specific immune response, which involves more specialized defenses against particular agents has two branches. These are known as cell-mediated and molecular immunity. Cell-mediated immunity or more simply, cellular immunity, is conferred by special types of white blood cells which directly engulf and/or chemically destroy pathogens or abnormal body cells. Molecular immunity involves the action of antibodies that circulate in the blood. With the help of blood proteins, these antibodies bind offending cells and molecules to which they have been sensitized by prior exposure, thus aiding in their elimination. So while we describe nonspecific versus specific immunity and cellular versus molecular immunity as if these were all independent processes, in reality they are intimately connected, coordinated, and often overlapping and constantly energetically communicating. From this point of view it is acknowledged that the whole is greater and infinitely more energetic in its workings than the sum of its parts.

Avoid seeking one protocol that you believe will do everything. Like I stated earlier, photon protocol should be one half of the treatment. Use multiple therapies that work together to support and power up the immune system and increase your odds for improving healing and recovery. It was recommended to use with the Photon the Cellect-Budwig protocol. We will discuss this in the next chapter.

Chapter 10

Other Alternative Methods

Cellect-Budwig

I am told the Cellect-Budwig cancer treatment is one of the strongest and fastest acting alternative treatments you will find. However, in this chapter, I will only be able to speak on the effectiveness of "The Budwig Therapy."

I contacted the National Cancer Research Foundation and requested information and permission to write about their product and its effectiveness on cancer. I spoke with Mr. Robert and was told to send him a short profile of myself to take before the NCRF. A couple days later, I received a message on my voice stating that NCRF was not interested in being in my book.

It's unfortunate I am unable to give my opinion about this product. If you want to know more about their supplement, research it on the internet. This protocol is based on two fast acting alternatives, "The Budwig and the Cellect." These two protocol's function to re-balance the body's biochemistry and the environment to a level that is correct for normal cells but is not conducive to cancer cells.

Budwig-Cellect is one of the few methods that does not produce inflammation and swelling. It is ideal for treating cancers where swelling could be potentially life-threatening.

The Budwig protocol utilizes a simple therapeutic dose of flaxseed oil and cottage cheese as a deceptively powerful cure for cancer and many other health problems. However, one can substitute other sulfurated proteins, such as yogurt or kefir, which requires higher amounts or whey concentrate powder.

Cottage cheese and flaxseed enhance oxygen delivery to the body's cells and thus increase cellular energy production. This will boost the cell function of the immune system to deal with the cancer or other unhealthy cells. It will enable the immune system to deal with microbial presence and toxins, and protect and energize the body's healthy cells. This may appear to be an unimpressive therapy, but surprisingly the potent effects on potentially fatal health issues includes heart disease and diabetes. Organic fresh fruit, vegetable nutrition, and sunlight are also recommended.

According to Dr. Budwig and those who studied and reported on this method over the last 50 years, there is a 90% success rate for curing cancer (lung, colon, breast, ovarian, brain, and others). This protocol has been used to treat arthritis, heart disease, arrhythmia, psoriasis, eczema, MS diabetes, respiratory conditions, stomach ulcers, liver dysfunction, IBS and other auto immune diseases.

Zeolite

Zeolite is a mineral that is one of the most powerful cancer cells killers. It is a remarkable volcanic mineral that has proven to be highly effective at destroying cancer cells in the body.

Zeolite comes in two forms: liquid and a powdered micronized form. Each is powerful detoxifiers and improves the alkalinity of the body. They are listed as cancer killers because Zeolite has the ability to activate the P21 gene which signals a cancer cell to die. Another important factor is that it has the ability to destroy the nucleus of cancerous cell.

A fourteen month study using liquid Zeolite showed that stage four cancer patients with a prognosis of about two months to live was given the liquid Zeolite. At the end of the study with 65 individuals, 51 were cancer free, six were alive but still fighting cancer, and eight died during the study. This is a 78% cure rate for terminal cancer patients. This cure rate versus that of the old orthodox treatments of chemo, radiation, and surgery is no comparison.

Zeolite is a negatively charged volcanic mineral that naturally attracts positively charged toxins to it and traps them in its cage-like structure. See below diagram.

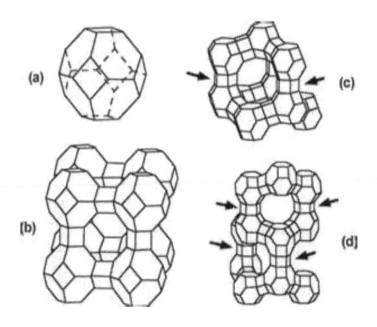

Zeolite's ionic charge turns slightly positive when it is full of the positive charged toxins it has captured. Normal cells have a neutral charge while cancer cells have a slightly negative electrical charge. So the slightly positive charged Zeolite molecule is now attracted to cancer cells.

Zeolite activates the P21 gene. The function of the p21 gene is to signal the cancer cell to die. This gene acts as a tumor suppressor as it controls the cell cycle progression.

Studies have shown that when cancer starts to grow, the cancer cell can turn off the p21 gene so that it can grow and spread without anything to stop it. This inactive gene allows cells that are diseased or not functioning properly to divide and spread. When the p21 is active, it allows your healthy cells to reproduce which strengthens your immune system and blocks movement of the diseased cells. There are no side effects because it specifically targets positive charged cancer cells.

Once the Zoelite is pulled inside the cell, the tri metallic part of the Zeolite molecule will destroy the nucleus and cytoplasmic organelles. In some cases, the cancer cells were destroyed in an outward burst of the cytoplasm by increased osmotic pressure. In other words, the cell wall and membrane collapse after the nucleus was destroyed and dissipated into the surrounding environment. Studies have shown that Cellular Zeolite works on the receptor sites, cell wall membrane, proteins, and surface chemistry of cancer cells only. An ordinary healthy cell is not affected.

Powdered Zeolite is not as proven as the liquid or Cellular Zeolite. It is not as purified as the liquid but it has cured cancer on its own. The powder tends to work more in the intestines and probably less in the brain. I recommend taking both at the same time because they may focus on different areas of the body. One container of the powder contains 450 grams, while a bottle of Zeolite contains 2.4 grams. The liquid does so much more with so little per drop.

There are other ways Zeolite fights cancer. It chelates and removes heavy metals, pesticides, herbicides, and other toxins from the body. The chelating takes place in an organized manner. First, it is attracted to lead, mercury, cadmium, arsenic, and other heavy metals. It then gets rid of the pesticides, herbicides, and plastics and traps viral particles, which stops production of viruses. Because it traps toxins in a molecular structure, it detoxifies the body without overloading the body.

Zeolite acts as a free radical scavenger and it boosts the immune system by increasing the CD4. CD4 cells are a type of lymphocyte (white blood cell) sometimes called T-cells. Zeolite also helps to normalize the body's pH levels. This product is labeled "generally safe" on the FDA's list.

Cellular Zeolite (liquid) is more activated and can capture more toxins than micronized Zeolite powder. They are both micronized, but made smaller in different ways. The powdered Zeolite is mechanically ground smaller. The heavy metals captured by the Zeolite is still in it so it's molecular structure is partially full and it can't detoxify as well as the completely empty cage-like the molecular structure of cellular zeolite.

The cellular zeolite undergoes several days of processing under high heat, also referred to as an acid bath. It is cooled slowly which rids the heavy metals and toxins and allows it to absorb ten to twenty times more toxins in each molecule than the powdered zeolite. An added plus is the liquid molecular structure is smaller and allows it to enter the bloodstream and into the cancer cell much easier.

Zeolite is nontoxic. It is a great detoxifier with an

amazing 78% cure rate of advance cancers. Can you imagine if the drug companies had this kind of effectiveness with one of their drugs? Every doctor in the world would be prescribing it.

Understand that although Zeolite may fight cancer, 12% of the patients in the study died. So it makes sense to fight cancer by dealing with as many of the underlying causes of cancer as possible.

The Zeolite protocol should be used with another protocol. As an extra protection, Zeolite on a regular basis, is excellent for preventing cancer. Now let's look at another effective cancer fighting alternative method.

CellAdam

Many years ago, CellAdam was developed by the Hungarian company, Biostemworld. This little known drug works by rebuilding the body's own adult stem cells and destroying tumor cells. For 25 years, it has been highly effective for treating cancer and proven to be the most effective when preventing early stages of cancer. It also impedes the malignant process, and has an analgesic effect in the hopeless stage of an advance tumor. Because of its natural composition, it has none of the hallucinogenic effects you get with morphine. The ingredients simply include a fatty acid complex extracted from soy and sunflowers.

CellAdam was founded by Adam Kovacs, a Hungarian researcher who devoted his life to finding a cure for cancer during the country's Communist era. Very few people know about this drug mainly because the literature is published in Hungarian for the international media, and the country's communist past and personal rivalries with the U.S. remain regardless of the fall of the Berlin Wall.

We have conflicts with large pharmaceutical companies. In the U.S., it's not only large pharmaceutical companies to contend with but the FDA, AMA and all of the other letter agencies who can't seem to find a cure for cancer.

Mr. Kovacs was a medical assistant and not part of the Hungarian medical establishment. The country's medical professionals, perhaps envious of his discovery, have been known to block his drug from wider distribution, but now it's reputation will allow it to be recognized by millions.

In fact check on eBay, they sale for $49.99. It is exported from the European Union, Hungary, and then brought to the U.S. They promise the seller will ship order within 2 days after receiving a cleared payment; no returns accepted. EBay guarantees that if you pay with PayPal you are protected 100%.

Biostemworld is partnering with a Catholic hospital in Rome, Italy to carry out human and animal research on the CellAdam drug. They would not disclose the order because negotiations are still continuing but the hope is that it will carry out more quantitative analysis to make the alternative therapy more viable. It can then be formally classed as a drug, have more credibility, and be distributed more internationally. The company is not looking to partner with the United States because the pharmaceutical industry is profit oriented and will attempt to discredit the drug.

What evidence is there that this drug really works? Well there is no shortage of testimonies in addition to the company's claim that it has a 75% success rate.

There is a case of a woman with lung cancer—the hardest kind of treatment—that was said to have been "incurable"-she went home to die. She tried Cell-Adam and within two months she was practically was healed.

CellAdam works by breaking down a shield that prevents cancer cells from communicating with the body's natural immune system, which allows it to kill the cancer cells. It assists the immune system to cure cancer by enhancing the body's system to be natural and allow a natural process to take over.

CellAdam's results have been mostly successful on patients who have cancer in the breast, lung, large intestine, melanoma malignant, and various obstetric tumors. It is a cancer prevention therapy and when used as a dietary supplement, it works by building up the body's adult stem cell count. Stem cells can decrease by as much as 80% in the course of a lifetime and can lead to signs of ageing, a weakened immune system, and diseases such as cancer. With CellAdam and its other nature based drugs, Biostemworld claims it can restore that count by as much as 75%. Not only does CellAdam prevent cancer but other diseases too.

Manioc

Cassava or Manioc Root is a fruit grown in various parts of the world. In the Philippines it is called Kamoteng Kahoy; Northeast India - Mogo; and in Africa - Mandioca, Tapioca root Kappa, and Manioc root. In South America it is cultivated as an annual crop. When it is dried to a powdery or pearly extract, it is called tapioca and the fermented, flaky version is called Garri.

Manioc is the third largest source of food carbohydrates in the tropics. Rice and maize are the first. In developing worlds, it's a major staple for over a half billion people. One of the advantages of this crop is its drought-tolerant and can grow in marginal soils. Nigeria is the world's largest producer of manioc, and Thailand is the largest exporting country of the dried manioc.

Manoic is classified as sweet or bitter. Bitter is preferred by many farmers because pests, animals and thieve are deterred. The Manoic roots are tubers that contain anti-nutritional factors and toxins and cyanide. If not properly prepared, they can cause acute cyanide intoxication, goiters, ataxia or partial paralysis.

These tubers are rich in starch and contain significant amounts of calcium, phosphorus, and vitamin C but are poor in protein and other nutrients. The leaves are a good source of protein but deficient in the amino acid methionine and possibly tryptophan.

Consuming manioc for prevention and treatment of cancer even in the terminally ill is not a new method. People in other parts of the world have known the power of this tuber and have been using it for years. For example, Dr. Cynthia Jayasuriya, who lives in Sri Lanka, revealed to the media recently that she experimented with manioc and was eventually cured of the cancer she had for a decade.

Dr. Jayasuriya cites the studies of Filipino Professor Manuel Navarro, one of the top oncologists in the world. Dr. Navarro said that manioc is an effective low-cost treatment to help reverse the growth of cancer. His advice is to take about a four inch average size manioc root, wash and peel off only the outer brown skin and blend it in a blender with two cups or 16 ounces of distilled water. Blend at high speed for about two minutes. Pour into a glass storage bottle and cool in the refrigerator. When it settles, all the dissolved starch will stay at the bottom and there will be nearly two cups of clear liquid on top. Drink one half of it (one cup) in the morning before breakfast and another cup in the early evening. The taste will be slightly bitter being that the base contains B-17. To counter the bitter taste, add fruit juice or flavor. On the first day, consume about four inches of the root and then increase it by half an inch the each day.

One day, a few minutes after taking the liquid, you may feel dizzy. Count this as your limit and tolerance level. The next day take an inch less.

Dr. Navarro said, "It kills cancer but be careful not to exceed the limit. It should not be given to children." He also said that it is not deadly "cyanide" and it is only Amygdaline B-17 which is somewhat similar in formula to cyanide, but lacks the "H" factor of the cyanide formula. Amazingly, cancer cells being non-aerobic, produce within themselves that missing "H" factor. Only the cancer cells are poisoned if they touch the B-17.

If you would like to eat the manioc root, boil with water to the top of the utensil. Old manioc must not be used and ginger should not be consumed even as ginger biscuits eight hours before and after consuming manioc.

Dr. Jayasuriya recounted some of the people she knew who spent very large sums of money for the treatment of cancer with injections and other forms of therapy but they suffered and die. Manioc is imported into the United States from Mexico.

Despite the public's support and growing interest in nontoxic and noninvasive alternative approaches, the medical establishment waged a fierce campaign against such therapies, labeling them quackery. Official medicine pours billions of dollars into narrow research that supports chemotherapy, radiation, and surgery as the major weapons in "the war on cancer."

That war has been a total failure in slowing the death rate. "It is a fraud", wrote Dr. Linus Pauling, two-time Nobel Prize Winner. Another Nobel winner, Dr. James

Watson, the co-discoverer of the DNA double helix, said it best. In 1975, he was asked what he thought of the National Cancer Program. He promptly replied and said, "It's a bunch of shit." Watson served two years on the National Cancer Advisory Board.

Gerson Therapy

The Gerson therapy was developed by Max Gerson M.D., a German doctor who migrated to the U.S. in the 1930's. Dr. Gerson experienced having migraine headaches, and believed the causes of these headaches were due to his diet. He developed a low salt, fresh crushed fruits and vegetable juice diet that was taken ten times a day. After a few months on this regime, he was cured of tuberculosis. He believed he could use the same therapy to treat cancer because cancer could not live in a body in balance with a functioning pancreas, liver, thyroid, and immune system.

The protocol called for detoxification of the body by taking 3-4 coffee enemas a day, which eliminates the dead cancer cells from the body. He also used supplements with various substances such as pepsin, Lugol's solution (source of Iodine) potassium, niacin, pancreatin (a digestive enzyme) and thyroid extracts, which are taken to stimulate organ function, especially the liver and thyroid.

Dr. Gerson also discovered that cancer patients had more sodium in their bodies than potassium. The sodium acted as a poison in the body because it is an enzyme inhibitor where potassium is the exact opposite and potassium is an enzyme activator. The purpose of fruits and vegetables in the diet is to correct the sodium and potassium imbalance. This in turn helps to revitalize the liver so it can rid the body of the cancer cells.

The patients documented by Dr. Gerson who were treated through the 1940's and 1950's lived in good health for many years. After passing away in 1959, Gerson's work is being carried on by his daughter at the Gerson Institute in Tijuana Mexico.

Urotherapy

It's been six years since one of my dear friends introduced me to a pain reliever for arthritis that guarantees the cancer would not return. He said, "It's called Urotherapy and you need to begin now." I asked what it required and when he explained it, I turned up my nose and gagged. Urotherapy is when you drink your urine as a medicinal aid.

He had been on it for years and was never sick. I listened to him boast about his experience but I thought to myself that this man was crazy drinking toxic waste. Years later, while researching alternative cancer treatments, I came across Urotherpy. The article was in *Nexus Magazine* and the title was "Healing with Urine Therapy."

The first sentence in the article was, "Urine is not a dirty toxic substance rejected by the body. The article goes on to explain that urine is a by-product of blood filtration, not waste filtration. Medically it is referred to as "plasma ultra filtrate." It is a purified derivative of the blood itself, made by the kidneys, whose principal function is not excretion but regulation of all the elements and their concentrations in the blood.

When you think of a healing therapy, you think of a therapy mentioned in this book, and not of a natural cure that our body creates on a daily basis. A therapy that has been proven, that will cure many diseases that plague us today.

You may feel a little nauseous when thinking about drinking your own urine but it has been clinically proven as one of the most powerful and successful substances we can use to heal our bodies.

For over a century, medical researchers have been conducting tests and it was proven that our own urine is a vital source of nutrients, vitamins, enzymes, hormones, and antibodies that cannot be synthesized or duplicated in any way. Urine has been used to heal heart disease, diabetes, infertility, asthma, auto-immune diseases, infections and many other ailments too vast to mention. Yet little information has filtered to the public as to its fantastic healing powers. We are just told that it is toxic waste that ends up in the toilet. But this therapy could mean the difference between life or death.

As an eleven year old child, I can remember when my mother was pregnant with my brother. She was approached by a company, one I can't recall the name, and was asked if she would sell her urine. She agreed. Every other day, a public health nurse would stop by to pick up the gallon jug which contained her urine. At the end of each month, my mother received a check but I never knew the amount. It must have been rather decent because she continued to squat over a jug for several months. Later in my years, I discovered that a pregnant women's urine was not considered to be just toxic waste.

Urine is an invaluable source of nourishment, but it is probably too controversial and not financially rewarding enough for the media, the medical industry or Big Pharma to talk about. And in no way will it be encourage or promoted as a potent healing therapy.

It has been proven through clinical studies that urine

has thousands of body chemicals and nutrients that reflect the individual's body functions. When these chemicals and nutrients are reused they act like vaccines, antibacterial, and antiviral and anti-carcinogenic agents. They also balance the hormones and act as an allergy reliever.

This treatment requires only your urine. Because it's like finger prints; no two urine samples are the same and no two urine samples contain the same components.

Don't dismiss this with a frown or a look of discuss on your face as I did some years back. This therapy has helped individuals with multiple sclerosis, colitis, lupus, rheumatoid arthritis, cancer, hepatitis pancreatic insufficiency, psoriasis; eczema, diabetes, herpes, mononucleosis, adrenal failure, allergies and more.

Individuals suffering from cancer can use the urine therapy in conjunction with one of the other therapies mentioned in the book. But, before you do, check with your health care professional. As I mentioned earlier, I am not a health care professional. All of these therapies have not been approved by the AMA or the FDA. Quite frankly, they won't be approved because they are not financially rewarding enough.

Let's look at how powerful urine is and how it heals a person with allergies. White blood cells referred to as "renegade" cells are believed to cause allergies. These renegade cells attack substances even when they cause no threat to the body. In order to cure the allergy these renegade white blood cells, called antigen receptors, are needed to correctly cure an allergy.

When these antigen receptors are reintroduced into the body, the body develops antibodies and these antibodies actually stops the allergic response. If you understand this process, you can see the ability to use this therapy to cure other diseases in the body including cancer.

According to BIOMEDX, there are two main ways to do urine therapy. This is not a complete discussion on how to use it, but simply an introduction.

The first way is to use your own urine in a homeopathic fashion. Collect midstream urine in a clean cup or container. This should be a clean catch, meaning the genital area (important for women in particular) has been cleaned beforehand. Add one drop of fresh urine to 1/6oz of distilled water in a sterile bottle. Cap and shake 50 times. Take one drop of this mix and add to another 1/6 ounce of distilled water and shake 50 times. Take one drop of the mix and add to 1/6 oz of 80-90 proof vodka which acts as a preservative. Place three drops under the tongue hourly until there is obvious improvement or temporary exacerbation of symptoms. As improvement progresses, lengthen the interval between treatments. After 3 days, suspend treatment to avoid pushing the immune system. Treatment is resumed if progress remains static or relapse occurs.

The second way is to place oral drops under the tongue then increase dosage as needed. Use fresh urine drops direct. For some cases, sub-lingual drops work well. (You should always use fresh urine immediately upon collection. You should not boil or dilute the urine in any way. You must use it in its natural form).

Start by taking 1-5 drops of morning urine on the first day. On the second day, take 5-10 drops in the morning. On the third day, take 5-10 drops in the morning and the same amount in the evening before bed.

Once you are accustom to the therapy, gradually increase the amount as needed to obtain results for your condition. As you use the therapy, you will learn to adjust the amount needed by observing your reactions to the therapy. You may work up to actually drinking an ounce or two at a time.

Paw Paw

The Paw Paw Treatment is only effective on newly diagnosed patients who do not have a fast-growing cancer or a cancer that has begun to spread. It is not recommended if you already had chemotherapy, radiation or surgery.

We all have unique body chemistry. An alternative treatment that works for your cousin may not work for you. Therefore, we must take the cocktail approach to prevent cancer cells from becoming resistant. Consider using two or three other alternative treatments presented in this book with the Paw Paw therapy.

Paw Paw comes from trees in tropical South and North America. Paw Paw's extract contains among other active ingredients, acetogenins, which modulate the production of adenosine triphosphate (ATP) in mitochondria of cancer cells. Acetogenins reduces the growth of blood vessels that provide nourishment to the cells. It also stops the growth of multiple drug resistance cells (MDR). Thus far, no other treatment, alternative or conventional has shown any effectiveness against multiple drug resistance cells.

Paw Paw has been found to be effective in depleting the cancer cells of their energy and preventing them from growing. It can reduce the risk of cancer as well it stop it from spreading.

Cousins to Paw Paw is graviola, guanabana and soursop. They are all fruits from a tree. However, the acetogenins extracted from Paw Paw are more active against cancer cells than the above three.

If we look at a tumor we find that approximately 2% of the tumor is made up of MDR (multiple drug-resistant) cells. Research shows that chemotherapy is not effective against these cells. When the first round of chemotherapy is introduced (if it is effective) cells that are not multiple drug-resistant do not show up in a scan. Since the tumor is made up of mostly MDR cells, the mass will appear to be effectively gone. MDR cells remain and start to multiply and regrettably a new tumor has formed, this time made up entirely of MDR cells.

When a second round of chemo is presented none of the cells will disappear on a scan because they are all MDR. The use of Paw Paw is the only cancer treatment that is effective by killing the MDR cells. One of the effects of PAW PAW is to reduce the ATP (adenosine triphosphate) energy in each cell of our body. Our cells have an electrical potential that effects how the cell processes energy producing substances mostly blood sugar and oxygen from our blood supply. ATP (adenosine triphosphate) used in cells as coenzyme are often called the "molecular unit of currency" of interacellular energy transfer.

By reducing this voltage level from 70 to 110mv to something in the 50mv region, normal cells can still function. Cancer and viral cells cannot process energy at this low voltage level; they would start to starve. This process is slower process than being poisoned which is why Paw Paw works slower than chemotherapy. When Paw Paw does not work, it is usually because it is not absorbed sufficiently to cause this voltage reduction. And if not, Cantron or Protocel may work. We will talk about Cantron and Protocel in the next section.

Paw Paw works by preventing cancer cells from feeding on glucose by reducing the ATP energy of the cells in our bodies. You must be careful when using it and know what to avoid, which will negate it's effect. Avoid taking high concentrations of Vitamin C, Vitamin E, Selenium, SOD, CoEnzyme Q10, and sea greens such as spirulina, algae, chlorella, and kelp. The vitamins found in fruits and vegetables will not affect the performance of Paw Paw because they are not in a concentrated form.

The following will affect the positive use of Paw Paw. Flax seed oil, hydrogen peroxide, PMB Techno, creatin, cellect, gensing, glutamine, taurine, rhodiol rhsea, d-ribose, magnesium, L-carnitine, resveratrol, collodial silver, pau d'arco with germanium, grapefruit seed extract, whey protine, iodine, IGF, enercel, MSM, cesium chloride, poly-MVA, hormone-blocking drugs, immunocal, and MMS (Miracle Mineral Supplement). Before using this treatment I recommend you do more research on your own, or speak with a health care professional first.

Side Effects

Cancer cells use 10 to 17 times more energy than a normal cell. Therefore, Paw Paw gravitates toward the cancer cell to cut off their supply of energy. If there are no cancer or high energy consuming cells in the body, Paw Paw will attack the fast growing cells in the intestinal system walls. It should not be used over a long period of time for individuals who do not have cancer. If you are a cancer patient, Paw Paw should always be taken with food otherwise it may cause you to be nauseas.

Cantron

It should be understood, you can't just select an alternative cancer treatment and suddenly the cancer is gone. Our bodies are different. What helped heal Johnny may not heal you.

One should consider the cocktail approach to prevent cancer cells from growing and spreading. For example, you may have to be do the Cantron Alternative Treatment and at the same time laetrile. Select a treatment you have faith in, do your research, and select the treatment you feel comfortable with.

After you have used the treatment for a while, and if you are not improving, the drugs your health care professionals have you on may be causing the treatment from being affective. That is why a successful cancer patient can prevent drug restive cells from developing by using three or more alternative cancer treatments. In other words, the "Cocktail Approach."

Cantron is a safe alternative cancer treatment. It has successfully treated people with a wide array of diseases for more than thirty years. However, it was sold under the names of Cancell and Protocel, which are different companies. Cancell and Protocel basically have the same formula with slightly different ratios of the same ingredients; both products having no dangerous side effects. Cantron has been tested and proven that not only is it anti-cancer, it is also strongly anti-viral and one of the most powerful antioxidants to have been tested.

It is effective against viruses including Herpes, Aids, Chronic Fatigue Syndrome, Lupus, Crohn's disease, Endometriosis, Fibromyalgia, and almost all auto-immune diseases. It has successfully treated Lou Gehrig's disease, Multiple Sclerosis, Muscular Dystrophy, Parkinson's Alzheimer's Leukemia, Rheumatoid Arthritis, and Scleroderma. Cantron has also been used to treat Heart Disease and High Blood Pressure. It has been noted that patients with cancer, high blood pressure, and clogged arteries who started on Cantron (cancer being the number one threat) found success with the treatments. But after the cancer was corrected, to the amazement of the patient, the high blood pressure was back to normal.

Cantron causes the cancer cell to self-destruct and literally explode. This happens by blocking the energy ATP, which is depleting the cancer cell of its energy until their membranes eventually cannot hold and the cell membranes burst apart. This process of bursting is called "lysing." If you continue to use Cantron, over time each cancer cell in a person's body will fall apart.

Chemotherapy drugs are used by most cancer doctors because it is a toxic substance and it has a profound toxic effect on fast-growing cells like cancer cells. The goal is to kill as many cancer cells in the body fast without killing so many of the healthy cells. Which in many cases will destroy the immune system and kill off too many of the healthy cells that eventually the person dies.

Cantron works differently and is non-toxic (cytotoxic). It presents a slower process that interferes with the natural energy production of the cancer cells in the body, causing the cancer cell to burst apart, while not interfering with the functioning of the normal healthy cells of the body.

The dead cancer cells are then processed out of the body as cellular debris.

Cantron starts working on reducing the energy production of the cancer cells immediately, but the cancer does not break down all at once. It starves the cancer cell of its energy, which may take weeks or months to make the body cancer free. This slow process allows the body time to process out the broken down cellular debris and remove it in a way that does not overwhelm the body's lymph pathways, the kidney's liver etc. which is the body's cleaning system.

It should be noted at this point that Cantron does not build the nutrient value or the immune system. One must follow a diet that is recommended for a cancer patient by their health care professional.

Bob Beck – Blood Purifier

The Bob Beck Protocol is one of the most effective of alternative treatments. It works a little different than the previous protocols in that it eliminates the microbes in the body which in turn gives the immune system the ability to concentrate on killing the cancer cells in the body.

The Bob Beck Protocol is classified as an electro-medicine protocol that builds the immune system. If you are in a weaken state, have only a short time to live or has been sent home because the doctors have destroyed your immune system, Bob Beck Protocol may not be the alternative treatment for you. It takes two to three months for it to really reach its maximum effectiveness. I recommend you use another alternative treatment along with the Bob Beck Protocol while it is working on the microbes.

Microbes

Microbes and the cause of cancer have been controversial for over a century. But it has been known and proven by outstanding physicians and scientist who have attempted to bring this knowledge of the cancer microbe to the attention of the public. Contemporary physicians like Virginia Livingston and physicians in the past such as Antione Bechamp and Wilhelm Reich who had brilliant cancer discoveries, were ignored and suppressed by the medical establishment.

Wilhelm Reich had legal problems with the FDA over the manufacture and sale of his orgone accumulators (also known as chi or life-energy) and the science of orgonomy. He was jailed and died in prison. Almost six tons of his books papers and journals were burned by FDA officials.

In 194, Livingston's book, "The Conquest of Cancer", caused such a controversy with the medical field that she was branded a quack. But years later, through the brilliant work of Livingston and other scientists not mentioned here, the mystery of cancer and the microbes that cause it were made public.

As I stated at the beginning of the book "everyone has cancer cells in their body." But why does a person get diagnosed with cancer and the other is not? Microbes and parasites enter the body and make their home inside organs of their choice. They enter through our food that is not cooked well, by the pollution, and many other external and internal sources.

These microbes rob the normal cells of the glucose needed in that particular organ. The microbes excrete toxic waste known as mycotoxins which are acidic and of no use to the cells. The cells of the organs that are invaded by the microbes are also robbed of nourishment and living in mycotoxins become weak.

When the organ becomes weak, the immune system becomes weak. When the immune system is weak it cannot kill the amount of cancer cells needed to prevent the cancer from growing out of control. Therefore, the cause of cancer is microbes and parasites that are in our organs or colon and blood stream which weaken the immune system.

The Beck Protocol cleans the blood of microbes within a few weeks. Originally, it was designed as a cure for AIDS, but it was noticed as a cure for cancer. Because of the time factor, there is a problem curing advanced cancer patients. It takes two or more months to be really effective in cleansing the body of the microbes that inhabit the blood and organs.

When the body has no microbes in the bloodstream the immune system becomes supercharged because there are no microbes and parasites to fight! The body can now make neuropeptides in larger amounts that get rid of the microbes. Once the microbes are destroyed in the cell the cancer is destroyed quickly.

MSM/LIPH

This protocol is based upon theory and solid testimonials by those that have used this treatment and were cured. The purpose of this protocol is to get massive amounts of oxygen and other microbe-killing substances inside the cancer cells, thus changing the cells back to normal.

This protocol also deals with inflammation and pain which is a factor of importance to a cancer patient. MSM (Methyl-Sulfonal-Methane) is considered to be organic sulfur. Before you purchase it, make sure it is from an approved authentic vender. Any product that is labeled MSM is not necessarily part of this protocol, which includes only a package that is labeled "Organic Sulfur." Remember, it must come from a reputable vender.

Another caution is do not take organic sulfur if you are on blood thinners or taking high doses of aspirin. If you are on chemotherapy, organic sulfur will make the chemo more effective and less damaging. Speak with your health care professional first before taking high doses.

It is recommended to take one tablespoon of organic sulfur two times a day. If you are on chemo, it is recommended you take one tablespoon three times a day.

Organic sulfur is a marvelous treatment by itself. pulls the oxygen from water and transfers it into both the cancer cell and the non-cancer cell. By adding LIPH, it makes the treatment more miraculous. The LIPH gets inside the cancer cells and kills the microbes.

The LIPH (pronounced Life) is a patent pending high pH combination of alkalinity and oxygen rich liquid silica. It does not need the MSM to get inside the cancer cells because the cells thinks the LIPH is nothing but water. Air is 21% oxygen, Water is 89% oxygen. The oxygen from air gets to the lungs, heart, and muscles, but the oxygen from the water is needed to get inside both the cancer cell and the "normal" cell in order to give them energy and to kill the microbes. By combining the MSM with LIPH its more effective. Make sure you drink plenty of water, one ounce for every pound of body weight.

For example, convert 150 pounds to 150 ounces, which is a little over a gallon per day. I know this sounds like a lot to drink, but a big glass every hour can enable you to reach your goal. Remember the water must be non-chlorinated with a half teaspoon of sea salt each day. Real salt is a specific brand that is rich in minerals. Minerals are really important for the transport of oxygen to parts of the body.

Iodine is essential. Use 5% Lugal iodine one to two drops daily in a small glass of water. Magnesium is also important in this protocol. You can get magnesium sulfate by taking a bath every other day in Epson Salt. Be careful not to take any prescription drugs, except for chemotherapy, two hours before and two hours after each time you use organic sulfur. This applies to two different four-hour periods during the day. For time released drugs, this protocol will not cause any side effects.

Beta Glucan

In fighting cancer, this remarkable system will protect and dispose of cancer cells if there is enough time to restore the immune system back to normal, which the answer to your recovery. Beta Glucan is referred and supported by many scientific journals compared to other immune system products that are hardly mentioned.

In order to recover, the immune system should be a number one concern. The following is how Beta Glucan works.

Beta Glucan is a safe and very potent biological response modifier that nutritionally activates the immune response through the Macrophage, Dendritic, and additional immune cells to yield various therapeutic effects. Microphages are important cells of the immune system that are formed in response to infection or accumulating damage or dead cells. Dendritic is a special cell that is a key regulator of the immune system, acting as a professional antigen-presenting cell (APC) capable of activating nave T-cells and stimulating the growth and differentiation of B-cells.

Beta Glucan is extracted from the yeast cell wall of Baker's yeast as Beta 1, 3/1, 6 Glucan, as a purified isolate with harmful yeast proteins removed and a processed to prevent reaggregation or clumping after exposure to water in the digestive sequence.

Beta Glucan nutritionally promotes normalization that includes regeneration of a suppressed immune response or a calming of a hyper response such as allergic reactions. Joined with proper diet, moderate exercise, adequate rest and reduced stress, the immune system can be maintained or as a goal returned to peak condition when nutritionally normalized with 1/3 Beta, 1/6 Glucan. An immune response performing normally is a key to success for anyone seeking a healthy life.

I would suggest chasing the Beta Glucan with a 4oz glass of water. Once the Beta Glucan goes down the esophagus, it passes into the stomach. Keep in mind that Beta Glucan is a complex carbohydrate, nature's armor, and that the stomach acid is not going to affect it. It will then pass from the stomach into the small intestine. The Beta Glucan micro particles are seen and consumed by M-cells or micro fold cells inside your Peyer's Patches which is located in your small intestine. Think of the Peyer's Patches as little Venus flytraps that physically reach up and grab these particles. They do not soak through the intestines. There is an actual grabbing of the particles which then pulls them through the lining of the intestine. Once inside these pockets, the particles are located in an area inside the intestinal wall called the GALT (Gut-Associated Lymphoid Tissue).

There are millions of immune cells sitting and sampling everything that comes through the gut and they are going to be attracted to the Beta Glucan, which holds the fingerprint of the yeast, yet it does not cause any of the reactions that yeast may cause. Once the particles are gobbled up and internalized, they will begin to travel throughout the body. They go to the lymph system through the lymph nodes and then into the liver, and soon into the kidneys, lungs, and bone marrow. This material is tracked throughout the body. As it travels, it breaks down these insoluble particles into water soluble molecules that are just the perfect shape and size to fit the CR-3 receptor aka an immunological cell surface receptor for a complement component which then activates the immune cells.

Side Effects

Beta Glucan is derived from Baker's Yeast, which is considered safe and non-toxic. All extractions from Baker's Yeast has been considered by the FDA as G-R-A-S (Generally Recognized as Safe) as a dietary food additive supplement.

Liver Flush

If you elect to use one of the alternative treatments before you get started it is suggested you cleanse your kidneys and liver. A thorough cleanse is important for a cancer patient or for any other disease prevention program.

A liver flush will help the body to get rid of gallstones in the liver, which will dramatically improve the digestion, get rid of allergies, back pain, shoulder pain, and many other illnesses that is directly caused by a polluted liver.

The flush will improve the immune system and over time will help it do what it is designed to do, which is to eliminate the bacteria, microbes, and parasites that steal energy from the cells in the organs by consuming their nutrients and empting their mycotoxins and other matter. These foreign bodies causes the organs to become weak and the immune system to not perform.

It should be noted that a liver flush does not automatically turn the immune system around. It takes a little time to re-energize the cells in the organs that were made weak by the microbes and parasites.

After the flush you should start at least one of the alternative treatments that you feel will be beneficial to you. The alternative treatment will kill cancer cells while the immune system becomes stronger.

When a person does a liver cleanse they should drink

plenty of water, a minimum of a quart a day. This is to flush out the mycotoxins and the dead microbes to prevent brain fog-a clouding of consciousness.

You can't do a complete cleanse of your liver when it has living parasites in it. You should get rid of the parasites before you start at least two or three weeks before the liver cleanse. Also, it is highly recommended that you complete a kidney cleanse before the liver cleanse. When these organs are working in good order (kidneys, bladder and urinary tract) the undesirable substances can be removed from the intestine as the bile is being excreted.

Dr. Hulda Clark wrote in her book, "The Cure for All Cancers" that three herbs will rid the body of over 100 types of parasites without getting a headache or becoming nauseous. They will not interfere with any prescription drugs as well. She said that these herbs are "natures gift to us." They are:

- Black Walnut Hulls (from the black walnut tree).
- Wormwood (from the Artemisia shrub).
- Common Cloves (from the clove tree).

These three herbs must be used together. Black walnut hull and wormwood kills adult and developmental stages of at least 100 parasites. Cloves kill the eggs. Dr. Clark said, "if you kill only the eggs, the million stages that are already loose in your body will soon grow into adults and make more eggs." They must be used together as a single treatment.

The following are the only essential herbs you will need for the first 18 days of the Parasite Program:

- One 30ml bottle of pale green Black Walnut Hull Tincture Extra Strength. This is 1 ounce or six teaspoons, enough for three weeks if you are not very ill.
- One bottle of wormwood capsules (each capsule with 200-300 mg of wormwood).
- One bottle of freshly ground cloves (each capsule with 400-500 mg cloves), or ¼ cup bulk powered cloves.

Dr. Clark stated that the two additional items that improves this recipe are ornithine and arginine. Parasites produce a great deal of ammonia as their waste product. Ammonia is their equivalent of urine and is set free in our bodies by parasites in large amounts. Ammonia is very toxic especially to the brain. By taking ornithine at bedtime, you will sleep better. Arginine has similar ammonia reduction effects but must be taken in the morning because it gives alertness and energy.

The following program was derived from Dr. Hulda Clark's book, "The Cure for All Cancers: Black Walnut Hull Tincture Extra Strength." On an empty stomach:

Day 1:   Take one drop in ½ cup of water.
Day 2:   Take 2 drops in ½ cup of water.
Day 3:   Take 3 drops in ½ cup of water.
Day 4:   Take 4 drops in ½ cup of water.
Day 5:   Take 5 drops in ½ cup of water.
Day 6:   Take 2 tsp. together in ½ cup of water.

You can stir the tincture with a fruit sauce to augment the taste. Drink it and hold for 15 seconds then swallow. If you are over 150 pounds, take two and one half teaspoon. If you are over 200 pounds take 3 teaspoons.

The alcohol in the tincture can make you slightly woozy for several minutes. Stay seated until you are alert and focused. If necessary, you can take 500mg of niacin amide to counteract the toxicity of the alcohol. If you feel slight nausea, get some fresh air or just rest until it passes. The capsules contain 200 to 300 mg of wormwood and should be taken with water.

Wormwood, before eating a meal:
   Day 1: Take 1 capsule.
   Day 2: Take 1 capsule.
   Day 3: Take 2 capsules.
   Day 4: Take 2 capsules.

Continue increasing dosage for 14 days until you are up to seven capsules a day. Take the capsules in a single dose or a few at a time. Do two more days of seven capsules each. After this, take seven capsules once a week for as long as you feel it's necessary; some take it for a lifetime. People with sensitive stomachs prefer to stay longer on each dose instead of increasing according to this schedule. Choose your pace after the sixth day.

Cloves, before eating a meal:
   Day 1: Take one capsule 3 times a day.
   Day 2: Take two capsules 3 times a day.
   Days 3, 4, 5, 6, 7, 8, 9, 10: Take 3 capsules 3 times a day.

After day 10, take seven capsules once a week. Take ornithine at bedtime for insomnia. If you do not suffer from insomnia, it may when you begin to kill the parasites in the body. Remember that to take arginine in the morning and daytime.

Chapter 11

Cheap Protocols

Cheap Protocols are inexpensive cancer treatments. In this book, however, I have been listing alternative methods that are affordable but yet a little costly such as Bob Beck Protocol, Cellect-Budwig, the Cesium Chloride etc. As the name implies, the Cheap Protocols are the least expensive treatments yet they are highly effective cancer treatments and can cure cancer by themselves.

I am fully aware that a great number of cancer patients do not have the financial ability to afford expensive protocols. These treatments can do the job plus help the person that has little finances. But first, there are some ground rules that I must cover.

If you are going to use an alkaline protocol use one at a time. For example, if you choose the Cesium Chloride you should not use it with the Kelmun Protocol (baking soda & maple syrup).

Some of highly alkaline items are: baking soda, kale, spinach, tomato, grapefruit seed extract, cesium, himalayan salt, Real Salt, garlic, wheatgrass, parsley, sprouts such as bean, pea, alfalfa, broccoli, avocado, high pH water (9.0 pH and above).

It is not a good idea to stop consuming all high alkaline protocols because in many of the other protocols the alkaline product is the key to its success.

Kelmun Protocol

The Kelmun Protocol is a combination of pure 100% maple syrup and free baking soda like Arm & Hammer. As mentioned in earlier chapters, cancer cells thrive on glucose. In fact they consume 15 times more glucose than a normal cell. With a mixture of maple syrup and baking soda, the maple syrup (glucose) acts as a Trojan horse. The cancer cell consumes the glucose but at the same time the baking soda is pulled into the cell which kills the cancer without harming the normal cells.

Alternative treatments using maple syrup, honey or molasses is designed to get microbe-killing substances inside a cell to destroy the cancer.

Key Ingredients

When you purchase the maple syrup make sure you buy the "Grade B" syrup. If you are having a problem finding grade B, you can use the darker "Grade A." One can substitute honey or molasses for the maple syrup as well. During this time, do not consume any type of "white sugar" because you want to get as much baking soda inside the cancer cell as possible.

The measurements are one level teaspoon of baking soda to three level teaspoons of 100% pure maple syrup. Using this measure, some people choose to mix several treatments together, but do not mix more than nine days at a time. Some will cook the mixture in a double boiler to make sure it is blended. Cooking is not necessary-it's a preference. After the mixture is complete, do not refrigerate. Keep at room temperature.

The dose amounts are important. If you are an advance cancer patient; take two, three, or four teaspoons of the mixture a day. If you are an advance cancer patient you can take as much as 16 teaspoons of the mixture a day, but only do this for a maximum of one week. Then decrease your dosage to four teaspoons a day for the remaining six weeks.

For an individual that is not an advance cancer patient, do not use more than one teaspoon of baking soda a day for 4-6 weeks, and do not extend treatment for more than six weeks at a time. After six weeks on the Kelmun protocol, take two calcium pills for three weeks and alternate back and forth as long as you wish. For example, six weeks on the Kelmun protocol then three weeks on two calcium pills then six weeks on the Kelmun protocol etc.

Again, remember to not combine a alkaline protocols. Only use one highly alkaline protocol at a time. Do not use the baking soda on the same day when using Cellect, Cesium, Calcium, or any highly alkaline product.

When mixing your baking soda and maple syrup, it is critical to differentiate between 1 teaspoon of baking soda and 1 teaspoon of the mixture. For instance, 16 teaspoons of the mixture is 4 teaspoons of baking soda and 12 teaspoons of maple syrup, and 4 teaspoons of the mixture is 1 teaspoon of baking soda and 3 teaspoons of maple syrup.

It is important to keep these numbers correct so you will not consume too much baking soda which will then elevate your pH level and cause Alkalosis, which is a serious condition. Alkalosis refers to a process reducing hydrogen ion concentration of arterial blood plasma (alkalemia). In contrast to academia (serum pH 7.35 or lower), alkalemia occurs when the serum pH is higher than normal (7.45 or higher).

Chapter 12

Epilogue

Not all individuals that choose alternative treatments survive from cancer. There are four reasons why.

First, after a cancer patient has suffered the chemotherapy, and radiation or surgery and their organs have been damaged, they then turn to an alternative treatment, and in most cases the alternative treatment was not strong enough to overcome the damage done to the body, and there just was not enough time left for the alternative treatment to work.

Second, when the patient elects the alternative treatment, he/she must treat themselves, and many mistakes can be made. The American Medical Association doesn't allow an orthodox doctor to treat a cancer patient unless it involves the old orthodox treatment (chemo, radiation, surgery.) If the doctor uses natural substances in treatment he runs the risk of losing his license.

Third, the NCI the FDA and other government agencies have suppressed the truth about alternative cancer treatments, and will not make public which alternative treatment is best for a particular cancer. With the lack of information many mistakes are made by the individual treating themselves.

Fourth, the media has "sold out" the public they are supposed to serve. They are caught up in the mass advertisement campaigns that Big Pharma provides. The media exists to serve their masters. Through these campaigns, the average person is totally brainwashed into believing that orthodox medicine is the only way to go. In fact, most of the public are not aware of any alternative treatment.

I once mentioned to one of my friends about how to build his immune system to kill cancer and other diseases in the body. He quoted the "talking points" that his health care provider told him which involved orthodox procedures. He said, "Who are you to override the advice from my health care provider?"

The four reasons I mentioned, are caused by a lack of integrity in the medical community through miss information, which is intentional and deliberate. If tomorrow, a legitimate cure for cancer was made known, how many Fortune 500 corporations would be out of business? A great number would close they're doors.

The lobbyists in Washington D.C. (who easily outnumber the seats in congress) fight hard to make sure these large pharmaceutical companies get what they want. These companies are known for financing political campaigns and influencing our legislators. We are lied to and the government is corrupt. It's all about the "Benjamins."

The cancer industry will do anything in their power to withhold lifesaving information about alternative treatments for cancer. They will publish deceptive statistics about orthodox cancer treatments, leading people in the wrong direction. These deceptive statistics only cause false hope and ultimately death to a cancer patient. It was Deepak Chopra who said, "There are more people living off cancer than those that have cancer."

As I stated in my disclaimer, the information I provided in this book concerning alternative methods are based upon my personal battle with prostate cancer. It is not meant to convey any impression that others should expect the same results, and I cannot guarantee that you will be cancer free in thirty-days like I was. Our bodies respond in different ways depending upon the extent of the cancer and where the cancer is located.

This information is critical if you or someone you know has been diagnosed with cancer. A physician should consult you about alternative methods; do not self prescribe. If your physician does not have an open mind, find one who would at least give one of these methods a try. A physician should respect your healthcare choice(s).

Today, 15 years later, my PSA is .015. When I was diagnosed with prostate cancer it was 26. These past years, I have been determined to share with you how I survived cancer. These alternative methods can heal your body with minimum or no side effects. They are natural so that your body can restore to its normal state.

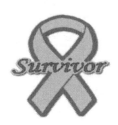

BOOKS/BIBLIOGRAPHIES
Armstrong, John W. *The Water of Life: A Treatise On Urine Therapy* (Random House Books – 2011)

Barron, Jon. *Lessons From The Miracle Doctor* (Kozy Books – 2015)

Bartnett, Beatrice & Adelman, Margie. L.M.T., C.N. *Miracles of Urine Therapy* (New Leak Distributors-1988

Blaylock, Russell L. MD. *Natural Strategies for Cancer Patients* (Kensington Publishing Corporation – 2003)

Clark, Dr. Hulda Regehr. *The Cure for Advanced Cancers* (New Century Press – 1999)

Clark, Dr. Hulda Regehr. *The Cure For All Cancers* (New Century Press – 1993)

Christy, Martha M. *Your Own Perfect Medicine: The Incredible Proven Natural Miracle Cure that Medical Science Has Never Revealed!* (Wishland Publishing – 1994, 1996, 1998, 2000)

Gala, Dr. *Auto-Urine Therapy* (Gala Publishers – 1990)

Humble, Jim V. *Breakthrough: The Miracle Mineral Supplement of the 21st Century* (Example Product Manufacturer - 2006)

Schreiber, Dr. David Servan. *Anticancer* (Viking/Penquin Group 2009)

Sircus, Dr. Mark. *Sodium Bicarbonate: Natures Unique First Aid Remedy* (Square One Publishers – 2014)

Chester F. Gaines

BOOKS/BIBLIOGRAPHIES (Cont)

Walters, Richard. *Options: The Alternative Cancer Therapy Book* (Paragon Press – 1992)

Wheeler, Virginia Livingston M.D. *Conquest of Cancer: Vaccines and Diet* (Waterside Productions – 1984)

INTERVIEWS
Floyd Jackson
Glenn Schwartz
Mildred Frankowski
Rodney McFarland
Sharlene J.

REFERRED ARTLCES
Business Week (September 22, 1986 issue about surgery, radiation, and chemotherapy)

Educate Yourself - The Story of Laetrile and Cancer (By Dr. Manners. - June 26, 2004)

pH of the Human Body is Critical for health (By Dr. Gary Tunsky)

REFERENCES
American Cancer Society (ACS)

National Institute of Health, Cancer Facts & Figures 2014 (Atlanta, Ga. 2014. Last Medical Review: 03/07/2014 Last Revised 03/31/2014)

WEBSITE CREDITS

Beta Glucan (http://www.betterwayhealth.com/blog/how-does-beta-glucan-work)

Bob Beck Protocol (www.cancertutor.com)

Biostem World (http://biostemworld.com/portal by Edward Pentin)

Ed. Skilling Institute (www.edskilling.com)

Energy Work (**www.energyworkinfo.com** by Rev. Barbara Clearbridge)

High pH Therapy-Cesium Chloride (**www.Essense-Of-Life.com or www.AbleVitamines.com**)

Photon Genius (www.cancertutor.com/about/EdSkilling)

WHERE TO PURCHASE PRODUCTS

Paw Paw is by Nature's Sunshine. Distributors in the U.S. are:

John Howlet, Nature's Sunshine Regional Manager (orders on-line in the U.S. or for ordering overseas). John is prevented by FDA regulations from making medical claims however he makes himself available to discuss protocols. Toll free number 1-888-523-1727.

New Beginnings in Health. Richard is not medically trained nor does he guarantee effectiveness. Toll free number 1 877-871-6262.

Green Black Walnut Hull tincture:
  Self Health Resources Center
  1055 Bay Blvd., #A
  Chula Vista, CA 91911
  Toll free 1-800-873-1663.
  Self Health Resource Center (Canada)
  14027 63ed St. Edmonton
  Alberta T5A 1R6
  Contact number 1-780-475-2403.

Wormwood capsules:
  Self Health Resources & Kroeger Herb Products
  805 Walnut St. Boulder, CO 80302

  Hanna's Herb Shop 5684 Valmont Road
  Boulder, CO 80301
  Toll free number 1-800-206-6722

Fresh Cloves:
  San Francisco Herb& Natural Food Co.
  1010 46th Street, Emeryville, CA 94608
  Contact number 1-510-601-0700

Note:

The author of this book has no financial interest in any company mentioned in this book or receives any financial returns from referring. The interest is solely to create a smooth transition for the reader as they enter into recovery.

The statements found within the pages of this book have not been evaluated by the Food and Drug Administration. If a product or treatment is recommended in these pages, it is not intended to diagnose, treat, cure, or prevent any disease. The information contained herein is meant to be used to educate the reader and is in no way intended to provide individual medical advice. Medical advice must only be obtained from a qualified health practitioner.

All information contained in this book is received from sources believed to be accurate, but no guarantee, expressed or implied, can be made. Readers are encouraged to verify for themselves, and to their own satisfaction, the accuracy of all information, recommendations, conclusions, comments, opinions or anything else contained within these pages before making any kind of decisions based upon what they have read herein.

Chester F. Gaines

How I Beat Cancer

Chester F. Gaines

50056034R00075

Made in the USA
Charleston, SC
08 December 2015